Slow Dancing
with the Devil

Slow Dancing with the Devil

A Son's Substance Use Disorder, a Mother's Anguish

SUSAN BARTZ HERRICK

Foreword by Angela Kennecke;
Afterword by Arun Gupta, M.D.

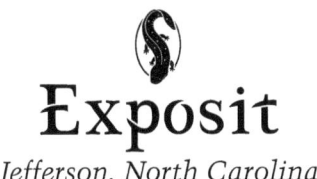

Exposit
Jefferson, North Carolina

ISBN (print) 978-1-4766-9389-7
ISBN (ebook) 978-1-4766-5155-2

LIBRARY OF CONGRESS AND BRITISH LIBRARY
CATALOGUING DATA ARE AVAILABLE

Library of Congress Control Number 2023054614

© 2024 Susan Bartz Herrick. All rights reserved

*No part of this book may be reproduced or transmitted in any form
or by any means, electronic or mechanical, including photocopying
or recording, or by any information storage and retrieval system,
without permission in writing from the publisher.*

Front cover images © 2024 Shutterstock

Printed in the United States of America

Exposit is an imprint of McFarland & Company, Inc., Publishers

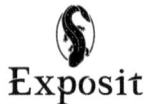

Exposit
Box 611, Jefferson, North Carolina 28640
www.expositbooks.com

To the memory
of my beloved son,
Robert "Luke" Paschal,
and all the other young people
who have lost their lives to Substance Use Disorder.
Your disease was ignored, as was your struggle.
Yet your lives have not been in vain.
You now inspire the heroes of tomorrow that fight
the stigma standing in the way of a cure.

***

Don't run away from grief, o' soul
Look for the remedy inside the pain
because the rose came from the thorn
and the ruby came from a stone.
       —Rumi

Table of Contents

Foreword by Angela Kennecke	1
Preface	3
CHAPTER 1. Once Upon a Time	5
CHAPTER 2. The Little White Pill	19
CHAPTER 3. The Price Tag	39
CHAPTER 4. Tough Love	65
CHAPTER 5. The Circle of Life	86
CHAPTER 6. A New Start	105
CHAPTER 7. The Unseen Enemy	126
CHAPTER 8. Broken Policies	154
CHAPTER 9. The Golden Years	182
CHAPTER 10. The Perfect Storm	213
CHAPTER 11. Dying for Change	239
Afterword by Arun Gupta, M.D.	245
Acknowledgments	249
Chapter Notes	253
Bibliography	263
Index	273

Foreword

by Angela Kennecke

Slow Dancing with the Devil is a gripping and heart-wrenching memoir that will take you on a journey through one mother's unimaginable struggle to save her son from the deadly grips of addiction. Susan Bartz Herrick's son, Luke, was just a teenager when he was first prescribed Oxycontin, a powerful opioid that pharmaceutical companies claimed was non-addictive. Little did they know this prescription would set Luke on a path to addiction that would ultimately lead to his tragic demise.

Through Bartz Herrick's powerful storytelling, you will be drawn into a world of pain, heartache, and resilience. Luke had so many factors working against him, from a horrific car crash that left him with a broken back to a medical mistake that only exacerbated his chronic pain. Despite his many struggles, what kept him alive for so long was his warrior mother, who refused to give up on him.

This memoir sheds light on the alarming failure of our nation's systems when it comes to addiction. From medical systems that prescribe addictive drugs to treatment centers that charge exorbitant amounts to insurance companies that often refuse to pay to the lack of access to medically assisted treatment, Bartz Herrick shows how our society is failing those who need help the most. As you read her story, you will come to understand that Luke's struggles could happen to anyone's child.

Slow Dancing with the Devil is a poignant and personal memoir that will help you recognize yourself in the story. You will develop more compassion and understanding for the way addiction ravages not only the person suffering from it but also all of those who love them. This book is a must-read for anyone seeking to understand the opioid crisis and the devastating impact it has on families across our nation.

Angela Kennecke is a veteran investigative journalist whose mission is to stop the stigma surrounding addiction and find solutions to the overdose epidemic. Her work took on a personal urgency the day she learned that her 21-year-old daughter, Emily, died of fentanyl poisoning. Kennecke is the founder of "Emily's Hope," a charity that offers help and treatment scholarships to families struggling with addiction.

Preface

The day I became my son's drug dealer, we both died, in a way. It is said that a mother would give her own life for her child. I would for Luke. A million times over. I wondered how many mothers would do the same to ensure their child would not die of a drug overdose or a rushed, unsupervised withdrawal. Yet that is precisely the situation my son and I faced. He depended on me. His life was in the balance. Saving him was all that mattered, and I was willing to risk it all.

Little did I know in 1991 that my son was born with numerous precursors to addiction. As the years went on, I was blind to the fact that I enabled his drug dependency. How could I know? Oxycodone was the wonder drug designed by Purdue Pharma to alleviate humankind's pain. Doctors passed it out like Pez, telling people it was only 1 percent addictive. That was a lie.

When the devastating devil drug took over my son's life after a near-fatal car accident, we were denied, by law, a legal drug called Suboxone that could ease his suffering and be a life-saving tool for recovery. Stigma and public policies forged in 1935 forced us to commit a felony by seeking it on the streets, as few medical doctors took the time to get the needed X-waiver to prescribe it.

Gone are the days when a single physician could provide all the needed medications for a patient. The unholy trinity now runs the legal drug cartel in America: insurance companies, the DEA, and nonscientific public policies. Physicians lost control and unknowingly led their trusting sheep to the slaughter. Hippocrates would be rolling over in his grave.

Society's understanding of substance use disorder, formerly known as addiction, is just as much to blame. Stigma still rules over science, calling SUD a moral deficiency instead of the chronic disease it really is.

The cultural image regarding an accidental overdose is that of a strung-out, undisciplined party animal. No one expects it could be an Ivy League student with a documented high tolerance who could not find reliable medical treatment and was forced to go to the streets to find relief from unrelenting cravings.

Yet that is what happened.

This book is a memoir. It reflects the author's present recollections of experiences over time. Some names and characteristics have been changed, some events have been compressed, and some dialogue has been recreated. Any resemblance to actual persons not giving their permission, whether living or dead, is entirely coincidental.

Chapter 1

Once Upon a Time

"Happy endings aren't always what we think they'll be."
—Snow White

When someone tells you who they are, believe them. On our very first date, Baxter told me he was a confirmed bachelor who would never marry again. On the other hand, I was husband hunting with visions of babies bouncing on my lap. Those facts alone should have ended the conversation with a handshake and well wishes, but they didn't.

Baxter and I met on a flight to Chicago. We hit it off immediately. He was 39, a chiropractic physician, wickedly funny, intelligent, handsome, and—most important—single. He told me right off the bat that he already had two sons from two separate unions and was not looking to go back down that road again. I was not deterred. Having a true gift for denial, I knew I could change his mind as he just hadn't met the right woman yet.

It was easy to fall in love with Baxter. The man made me laugh, and his intellect kept me engaged. We had fun together even though our dates always ended up at a bar with him drinking an excessive amount of alcohol. That by itself was a warning flag but one I did not heed. When fear and desire drive one's bus, one tends not to see the danger signs looming in plain sight.

After a few months of dating, I thought it was time to muster up the courage to see if he thought we had a future together. My biological clock was ticking louder than Big Ben. At age 30, I knew there was no time to waste. Gathering up my courage after two weeks of role-playing the conversation, I dove into the dark waters of his painful past.

"Two years," I announced insistently after he downed his tenth beer of the evening. I waited that long, hoping it was enough to wear down his resolve. His silence gave me the courage to go for the second hardball pitch. "That's it. We'll date for two years; I'm gone if you can't commit by then."

Baxter, fidgeting with his cigarette, sat quietly on his bar stool before stoically replying, "Make it four, and we'll get married."

"Four? Seriously?" I stammered in disbelief, projecting my disappointment into my water glass.

"Your choice—take it or leave it," he said with a playful grin, reaching into his back pocket and tossing down a brochure for a resort in the Bahamas.

I am ashamed to say I could be bought.

*****

We had started dating long distance as I lived in Chicago and he was in North Carolina. Circumstances were on our side. After receiving an MFA in theatre two years before, I took a job as a flight attendant so I could audition on both coasts and see the world before settling down. I could hop on a plane anywhere in the world for pennies on the dollar. Baxter had his beloved four-seater airplane and was a gifted, experienced pilot. We were quite the jet-setting couple meeting in different cities across the country. It indeed was a fairytale romance.

After a year of dating, Baxter came to see me in Chicago for the weekend, flying commercial this time as he'd sold his old airplane and was waiting for the delivery of his new forever dream plane, a Mooney M20J—the Porsche of the skies.

On this particular flight, Baxter was seated next to the assistant administrator of a psychiatric hospital and drug treatment center in Fayetteville. They instantly became drinking buddies and thus best friends. It came up in conversation that the hospital was looking to hire someone in its public relations and marketing department. Specifically, they wanted a trained public speaker. Baxter's ears perked up, and he told the administrator I had a lot of experience in the field. Five cocktails later, I was hired sight unseen. Two weeks later, I willingly hung up my wings and moved to North Carolina to be close to him and start a new career.

My new job was diverse. Primarily I was marketing multiple departments of social services in the state for referrals and making radio and TV commercials. My favorite role, however, was lecturing at civic organizations about substance abuse and other mental health issues as the hospital's clinical staff was busy dealing with patients. Even though the mental health field was new to me, I could research and learn—which I did.

Six months into the job, HR called me with some disturbing news. They mistakenly thought my MFA was somehow related to mental health. Oops—their bad! They loved my work, however, and knew I had put hours of research into each topic, so they gave me the option to keep my job and go back to school to get a Master of Social Work or a Ph.D. in psychology.

Really? Ugh. Yet I had no choice if I wanted to keep that good-paying job. I started looking at programs. Online classes were not yet available, but distance learning was gaining momentum. After searching the Internet, I found an Ed.D. program in human development and proposed it to HR. The hospital administration accepted my proposal, and I started gaining credit hours for the research I had already been conducting for my lectures. Off I went into the community, lecturing about the evils of alcohol and drugs, touting that prevention was the only cure. I'd meet Baxter for dinner in the evenings before going home to study.

Working at the psychiatric hospital brought the harsh realities of mental health disorders out of the news headlines and directly into my daily encounters. One could not just turn the page and ignore the suffering anymore. Screams had faces. Broken minds had names.

Addiction was recognized as a disease only by a few medical organizations. The efficacy of the 28-day treatment programs revolved around the amount of insurance people had. More often than not, 28 days were insufficient to maintain sobriety once the patient was discharged.

When the patient count was low, I would help in the children's ward, getting exposure to the emotional effects of child abuse. Sadder yet was watching the children being released right back into the same environments that put them there in the first place. Again, it was an easy call, as they were sent home when their insurance ran out.

As a part of my education, I also had to sit in on case study meetings with the clinicians as they discussed treatment for their patients.

I gasped one day when the alarms went off as we witnessed a patient breaking out of the front door with a host of white jackets in hot pursuit. As quickly as everyone looked up, they went back to their meeting. One psychiatrist saw my distress and made the offhand remark, "It's not a crisis."

"What do you mean it's not a crisis?" I blurted out in utter dismay.

He stoically replied, "The definition of a crisis is asking, 'Will a child die due to this action?' If the answer is yes, it's a crisis. If not ... meh."

We all returned to the matter at hand, but inwardly I was shaking. My upbringing had not prepared me to deal with the darker side of life. There was a stigma surrounding people who had mental health disorders or were addicts; they were hidden from public view. Any mention of having once seen a psychiatrist could hinder employment in the public marketplace. Depression was considered a lack of faith in God or at best a sign of weak character. Every employee at the hospital even had to sign a privacy disclosure forbidding us to identify any patient. Failure to comply would result in instant termination. Ignorance was bliss.

*****

Public policy was not helping anyone understand the true nature of addiction, as the call to action in the media was "Just Say No." Even though the current *DSM-III* stated addiction was a disease, its new definition fell grossly short of the reality that would remain hidden for decades.

The *Diagnostic and Statistical Manual of Mental Disorders* (*DSM* for short) is the handbook used by healthcare professionals in the United States and much of the world as the authoritative guide to diagnosing mental disorders.[1]

In 1986 the *DSM-III* spelled out the chief symptoms of addiction as "a compulsion to use a psychoactive drug, the loss of control over the use of the drug, and continued use despite adverse consequences." In other words, being addicted was your own fault, a true moral ineptitude. There was no mention of stages of the disease or precursors, genetic or otherwise, that took the onus off the individual and allowed them to have proper care and respect. Stigma ruled the day. Addicts were lowlifes who were devoid of self-control and had moral deficits. That was the consensus of society at the time, including me.

When the *DSM* first came out in 1952 from the American Psychiatric Association, it had many concepts and suggestions that would be shocking to us today. [para] *"Infamously, homosexuality was a 'sociopathic personality disorder.' Autistic spectrum disorders were a type of childhood schizophrenia. These diagnosis thoughts were circulated as medical truth until 1973."*[2] Yet if the *DSM* said it, it was considered scientific truth.

My eyes were opening to the agony of addictions, yet they were slamming shut to what was happening in my personal life. Many of my colleagues knew Baxter and cautiously asked me if I thought his drinking was a problem, even suggesting he was a functional alcoholic. As an unsuspecting codependent, I maintained that he had a high tolerance and not a substance abuse problem. After all, alcoholics were bums in the gutter, and Baxter was anything but. Denial is a significant factor in dealing with family members of alcoholics and addicts. Even though my eyes were slowly opening to the concept of people self-medicating emotional trauma, I could not see the forest for the trees.

After three and a half years of dating, I finally had the guts to give Baxter the ultimatum—marry me, or I'm leaving. We were living together even though I had my own apartment. I never dreamed he'd turn me down, but he did. He asked me to stay on as his girlfriend. That is all he had to offer. Devastated, I walked out. I still wanted my house with a white picket fence and a family.

After three months of separation, Baxter called late on a Friday night. We talked casually at first but quickly reminisced about fun memories and we decided to go on a date the following evening.

In short order, he confessed he was devastated without me and tried to lure me back with two fur coats, a Rolex, a big house, and diamond earrings. Oh, and a marriage proposal complete with a five-carat diamond ring.

"Not so fast!" my heart shouted. Even though I loved him dearly, I went away for the weekend to think about it. *Could he really change?* Probably not, as I knew I forced him into buying into my dream. But it was all in front of me, loaded with gold and glitter to entice me past my better judgment. Ashamedly I was a sucker for the good life. In short, I convinced myself my love could change him in time. After all, he swore once that he would never marry again.

In a last-ditch attempt to get what I wanted, I wrote a three-page letter of demands. The trinkets were all well and good, but I needed more. I wanted a husband who *wanted* to be married—a family man who also wanted a child. I wanted to settle down in a home and make a family. The white picket fence itself was optional—but nothing else.

After skimming my letter, Baxter agreed to my demands, assuring me he wanted the same things. He even told me he'd consider having more children in a few years.

Done! That is good enough for me!

Three months later, on December 29, we were married. Six months later, I became pregnant. Much to my surprise, Baxter took the news with grace and a smile. He and his eldest son Worth promptly went out drinking to pick out baby names. They came home five hours later announcing the baby would be a girl and her name would be Laura. I just shook my head. Three months later, amnio results told us it would be another boy. I hesitantly asked Baxter if he was disappointed.

"You can never disappoint a man with a son, sugar," was his reply.

I was relieved and started thinking of names, announcing to all that I would have the final say. Robert after my father. Luke after the apostle who was a physician in the Bible. We agreed to call him Luke.

After finding out I was pregnant, I left my hospital position. The previous summer, I had been in a theatrical play and the department chair at the university in town had seen the production. He was impressed enough to offer me an adjunct teaching position. I accepted without hesitation. I loved the mental health field, but my heart was in the arts. It also meant fewer hours with a lot of time to prepare for my precious son.

*****

Robert "Luke" Paschal was born at 11:06 a.m. on February 11, 1991—Apgar rating 10; seven pounds, 11 ounces with all 10 fingers and toes. My heart was full. Baxter brought him around to see me after the C-section. Luke was fussing up a storm.

"Luke—it's Momma," I whispered softly, holding out my finger.

Chapter 1. Once Upon a Time

Instantly he stopped crying and grabbed on tightly, his big black eyes desperately blinking to find me. Our forever love had begun as he was laid over my heart.

My mother came down from Chicago to help me get settled. While sitting in the kitchen one morning, I was overtaken by an intense yet frightening love for this tiny human being. While rocking him in my lap, I pondered my heart's profound, unexpected changes. Life was no longer about me. Instantly, every cell in my body focused on this tiny black-haired beauty in my arms.

"Momma, how long does it take for this feeling of complete vulnerability to go away?" I gasped, trying to take it all in.

She paused, sipping her tea, and replied softly, "When it happens, honey, I will let you know."

My mother left two weeks later, and I knew I'd have to figure motherhood out alone. Because I was an older, educated woman, I read up on motherhood. Books tell you everything, right?

The book *What to Expect When You're Expecting* by Heide Murkoff was popular. I read about a mother who did not get a full night's sleep for two years as her child needed to nurse every three hours. My heart went out to her. "Poor dear," I thought. Little did I know I would break her record and not get a good night's sleep for the next four years and then some.

Luke was cute as a bug from the day he was born. I'd always get stopped by people oohing and aahing over his physical beauty. Thus my pet nickname for him: "Bug." He also never slept—or so it seemed. He nursed every hour and a half and needed constant motion or he'd wail as if being tortured. That schedule is a good reason to have babies in your 20s. However, all that fatigue melted when I looked at that little face and saw those tiny arms reaching up only for me.

We had a beautiful cradle next to my side of the barely-used bed. I'd nurse Luke and lay him down, hoping for a few hours of sleep. No such luck. He'd fuss up a storm the second he sensed he was alone. Exhausted, I'd pick him up to snuggle as we fell asleep in the big bed.

Luke's erratic sleeping habits grew over the years. Little did I know these were signs that he suffered from neurological conditions that would chart the course of his entire life. He needed to be in constant motion even when he was awake. As a baby, he had to be in his crank-up swing or bouncing in his airplane that hung from the door casing. He also had to be in constant motion in the stroller, which made shopping a challenge as I'd have to circle the dress racks or grocery aisles to get what I needed. He'd wail if I came to a standstill.

Settling him down for a nap required a car ride or putting him on the back of my bike strapped in his seat. Carefully and oh so cautiously, I'd unstrap him and carry him up to his room. If he woke up, we'd have to start the process all over again. He stopped taking naps at age two, which nearly did me in, as I desperately needed them. Trying to outsmart and keep him safe, I'd put on children's videos and stack cardboard bricks in front of the playroom door while I crashed. Most days, it worked like a charm.

Bedtime was also a challenge. Most children go to bed at 7 p.m. Not Luke. Even as a baby, it was around 10. I'd lie down with him and sing him to sleep, but three hours later, he'd be awake, screaming. Lovingly I'd walk the floor with him or rock him for a good hour until he fell asleep. If I didn't stay with him, he'd wake up again within an hour. To avoid sheer exhaustion, we played musical beds between Luke's room, the guest room, or Baxter's and my bed. Even though we all went to sleep in our respective places, I never knew where I'd wake up. I just knew Luke would always be snuggled close. It was a roll of the dice where we'd end up in the morning, but it was the only way for the three of us to survive. I'm sure Dr. Spock would have pulled my motherhood privileges, but he wasn't the one sleep deprived.

Night terrors were also becoming more frequent and gradually accompanied by sleepwalking. At first, we thought he was just being cranky until we tried to make sense of his rantings. It was then apparent that he was sound asleep. I was the only one who could calm him down with soft singing. He'd focus on my voice and let me wrap him up in my arms and carry him back to bed. One night in the dead of winter, we heard some racket from the dogs and saw him standing outside in the backyard pretending to direct traffic. Mortified, we grabbed him and promptly put tall locks on the doors and installed an alarm system in the house.

Multiple sources state that approximately one in six children suffers from night terrors. They are most common in children between two and four but can happen in children up to age 12.[3] Most children outgrow night terrors by the time they reach puberty. Luke did not. His night terrors continued throughout his life, although they decreased as he entered his late teens. It was harder to comfort him at that age, and more than once, I got hurt, once almost knocked out, trying to calm him. I asked him what he saw during these events when he was older.

"Dark shadows in the corner. They are scary, and they are after me," he would reply. How I wish I had known of magnesium's calming effect on the brain back then.[4]

*****

We first saw Luke's intellectual potential when he was three and a half. While we were driving directly into the bright setting sun, he piped up from the back seat, "Momma, is Jesus called the Son of God because he shines brightly in our hearts like the sun does in the sky?" We all just looked at each other, dumbfounded. Mom just smiled and scheduled educational testing at her school on our next visit to Chicago.

No one was shocked at the numbers. Two separate IQ measurement tests had him around 143. He was well above the norm in cognitive development, with scores in the upper range of characteristics associated with giftedness. The best area of response was that of specific academic abilities. Of note were responses related to his tendency to ask in-depth questions regarding subject areas of interest and his ability to demonstrate significant knowledge of those interests, such as subjects requiring abstract thinking like mathematics, the sciences, and philosophy. Luke threw away the LEGO instructions during the test and created a unique contraption that surprisingly worked with trap doors and complex side parts.

Some observations were cause for concern, such as an unusually high level of anxiety. Luke would need extra time when taking tests as he panicked at being under pressure to perform. He also desired perfection in these subject areas, which caused more anxiety. Lastly, and of most concern, OCD tendencies and acute ADD were a possibility. Only a physician can diagnose these neurological disorders, so the wording of these conditions was nebulous, but the test administrator's information gave us a heads-up.

Luke's grandmother was naturally concerned and wanted him to get the best education. She was a well-respected educator in gifted

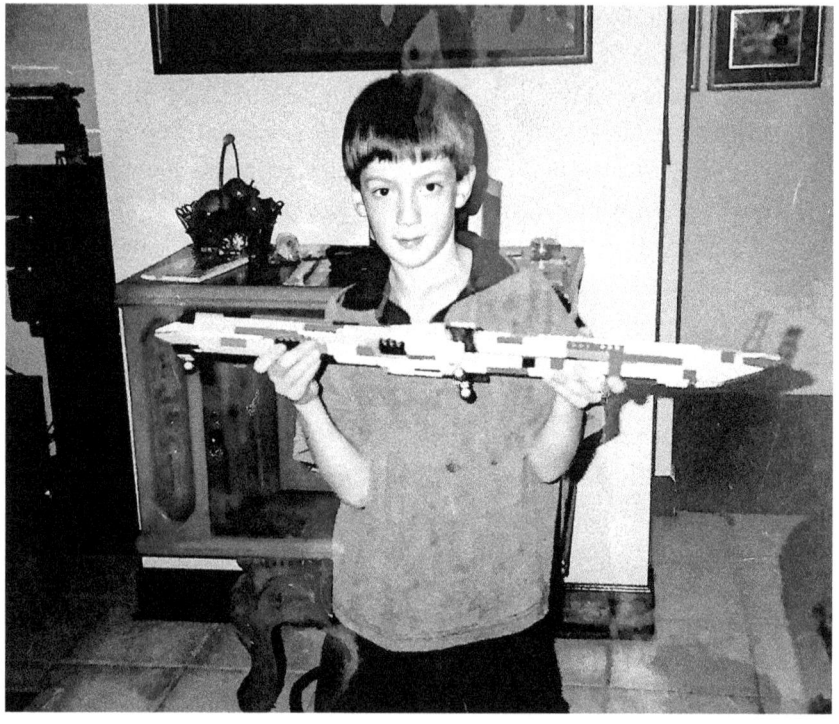

Luke Paschal, age seven, with his original Lego creation.

education and encouraged us to move to Chicago so Luke could go to one of her schools for the gifted. That, of course, was an impossibility.

As Luke went on in school, the problems began as my mother predicted. His first two years were successful because he had teachers who understood that not all children learn the same. He was allowed to read underneath his desk or upside down in the corner. He had trouble with reading comprehension yet could have intellectual conversations with adults that would make your eyes cross.

Much to my surprise and delight, Baxter tried to be a good father. He loved his little boy and seemed to be happy to be able to finally raise one of his three boys from scratch. And Luke adored his daddy. Every Halloween, they would dress up in matching costumes. Going to Toys"R"Us was a weekly adventure reserved for them alone. Sometimes I thought Baxter behaved as much like a kid as Luke as they both had such fun playing with LEGO sets or computer games. I remember the day Baxter almost cried when Luke told him he didn't want to go to that "kids store" anymore but wanted to go to the "Daddy store"—aka Best Buy. Flight simulators then became the new obsession, as well as space travel. When Luke was nine, they visited the U.S. Space & Rocket Center in Huntsville, Alabama, for father-son space camp. The picture of them together, in uniform, was always on Luke's dresser.

Our life looked beautiful on the outside. Money was good. We had a large home in a nice neighborhood, an airplane, and a big Mercedes Benz. Baxter even fulfilled one of his dreams and bought a condo on the 34th floor of a building on Oak Street in Chicago, close to where Grandma and Grandpa lived, where we would frequently go on the weekends. We'd take side trips to Texas for the Mooney airplane convention, go to the Caribbean, or follow Duke sports around to wherever the teams were playing. Luke always traveled with us. The problem was that his father's drinking came along too and Luke was noticing.

"Why does Daddy's breath smell so bad in the morning, Mommy? Why is Daddy so mean the day after he 'works late'?" Luke's questions were unanswerable. How do you explain detoxing to a four-year-old?

It turned out I didn't have to. It was 2 p.m. on a Saturday. While folding laundry, I saw Luke sneak into the kitchen. Thinking he would grab a snack, I stayed my course folding the socks. Suddenly I heard rattling and froze. He was taking the remaining four beer bottles from the refrigerator and putting them in a grocery bag. My first instinct was to reprimand him as I thought he was taking them up to his father. My rage built like Mt. Vesuvius as I prepared my speech to both father and son. Much to my surprise, Luke stealthily walked through the back door, dragging the bag with the bottles behind through the pine straw. *Oh my God, is he going to drink them?* Struggling to put on my shoes to go after him, I saw him pick up his small shovel and bury the beer 15 feet from the house. Still stunned, I watched from behind the door as he skipped back to the house and ran to the playroom announcing, "Let's play, Daddy! No more beer in the house—just me!"

My heart sank. I promptly called my mother for advice.

*****

Thank heavens for my parents' love and devotion. Five years after my father passed away in 1983, my mother married a man named Joe. Mom had known him from the church where my dad had been the head pastor. I had been in the same class as Joe's eldest son and had known the family well for more than 25 years.

Joe was a good man and quickly earned the title "Papa Joe" for me and "Grandpa" for Luke. He filled the hole in my heart from losing my dad when I was 28. Joe was Luke's only living grandfather. I found myself putting a great deal of expectation on Grandpa to be a strong male influence on Luke. Grandpa took Luke to the park and to play putt-putt and he taught Luke to swim and fish. They were buddies from the get-go.

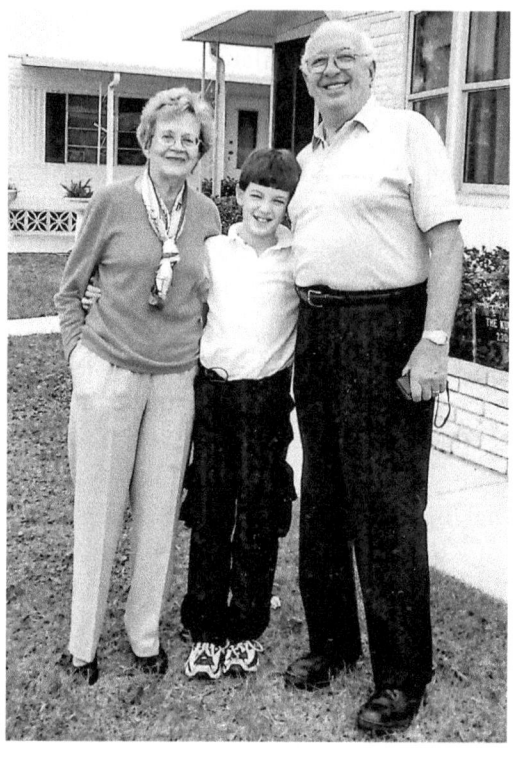

Grandma, Grandpa Joe, and Luke, age nine. He loved them so.

My mother was my best friend and confidant. I had a great deal of respect for her professionally also. She was a celebrated educator who founded two schools for the gifted in the Chicago area and operated her own health and wellness business as a Shaklee distributor. Even in her 70s, she gave the Energizer Bunny a run for his money. And she was wise.

Luke was my mother's favorite grandchild, without question. She loved all her grandchildren deeply, mind you, but Luke was the one who came running into her arms and wept whenever she would leave, as did she. My mother was allowed to be a part of his life and dove headlong into ensuring he had all the tools to succeed. Regrettably, Grandma and Grandpa lived hours away, and we would never have enough time together.

*****

Unfortunately, substance abuse does not stand still and in time drives a wedge between the most loving couples. Decisions become clouded. Stonewalling sets in where there was once laughter. As the years progressed, Baxter and I drifted apart. He purchased a minor league basketball team and was busy building new practices despite a failing economy. I was busy trying to salvage my son's education.

Grade school was a challenge for Luke. Despite his high IQ, he could not focus, and his reading comprehension was below grade level. Determined to find answers, I took him to the pediatrician. After a few hours of testing came the results: ADD and Tourette syndrome—both neurological misfires in the brain.[5]

Tourette's is an inherited neurological disorder. It begins in childhood and is characterized by the presence of multiple physical motor tics and/or vocal tics. Luke presented primarily with motor tics, not vocal. He quickly learned to try to conceal them with shrugs or other diversions as he was getting picked on and laughed at in school. These tics dissipated with age but never totally went away. In time Luke got very creative at masking them, as most afflicted learners do.

The doctor gave me a choice to treat one ailment or the other, as the medications for one of these disorders would cause the other to get worse. I chose to treat his ADD. The drugs of choice for his ADD were Adderall or Haloperidol, sold under the brand name Haldol for Tourette's.

I knew Haldol from the psychiatric hospital. It is an antipsychotic medicine used to treat schizophrenia and has terrible side effects. That was not going to be an option! I opted for Adderall against my mother's wishes. She wanted me to take the natural approach using B-complex vitamins and chewable magnesium, but I didn't listen. I wanted clinical proof they worked; there wasn't any then. If only I had listened.[6]

Adderall certainly helped Luke focus, and his grades instantly went up. His Tourette's, however, became substantially worse, and he only slept three to four hours a night.

Adderall is known to increase the activity of some neurotransmitters, especially dopamine. Over time, the changes in dopamine activity can impact the brain's reward center and alter one's ability to experience pleasure without chemical support. Children's brains are in a critical developmental stage, and neuropathways are being set in place.

People of all ages can get used to these high dopamine levels over time and feel dependent on the drug. If only I had known Adderall could be a gateway drug to addiction.[7]

You will not find many medical doctors agreeing with that last statement, as most studies did not support that claim then. The pharmaceutical companies that run the studies may be to blame. But do a Google search on drug treatment centers, and you will find Adderall listed as a significant addiction they treat. After all, methamphetamine (meth) and Adderall, an amphetamine, are related. Let's just call them kissing cousins.[8]

Luke finally begged me to get him off the medication. After a year of Adderall, I trusted my mom's instincts, ported to the natural way, and apologized to them both. His ADD returned, but he slept in a much better frame of mind.

But all was not well on the home front. Rumblings of disaster were echoing through the halls. As much as I condemned Baxter for his drinking, I also had to look at my increasing wine consumption. It was easier to drown our problems than deal with them.

Chapter 2

The Little White Pill

"Pain could be killed. Sadness could not, but the drugs did shut its mouth for a time."—Colson Whitehead

Two events in 1991 changed my life forever: the birth of my son Luke and the practices of the Sackler family. The New York–based family company rebranded from a little-known pharmaceutical company called Purdue Frederick to become Purdue Pharma and began developing a revolutionary new drug—Oxycontin. Unfortunately, my son was predisposed to have a contentious relationship with the poisonous Basilisk long before the world knew of its lethal nature. Tragically, I did not know, and we fell into its deadly trap as the years ensued.

My fairytale life came to an end in 2001. Creditors were calling daily. The grocery store denied my credit cards. There was no health or auto insurance. The airplane was still in the hangar, yet the house was in foreclosure—all unbeknownst to me. In the blink of an eye, we had lost everything. Baxter's overextended investments, my denial of any problems, and a failing economy bankrupted us. His attempts to hide everything from me and the IRS resulted in disaster. In a drunken explosion one night, he watched his life disintegrate before his eyes as the truth emerged through a summons. That event finally cracked open my denial, revealing a chasm no Band-Aid could cover. It was time to take a stand.

"Marriage counselor and financial counselor, or I am gone!" I sternly told Baxter the following day in the bedroom. It was not a threat but a calm, clear statement of fact. "And get rid of that airplane so we have a place to live!"

"Over my dead body!" came his exhausted response. "I can work this out—trust me. We'll rent an apartment for a while, but I am never getting rid of my plane!"

He then packed his bag and flew to a Nebraska football game for a long weekend, leaving Luke and me only $20 in cash for food or emergencies. My heart sank. I watched my love for him walk out the door when he did.

Baxter's priorities cut me like a knife. Unfortunately, Luke was standing in the corner of the bedroom and overheard everything. I finally faced the heartbreaking reality that my fairytale dream was nothing more than a delusional fantasy. At that moment, a flash of clarity told me it was time to move on.

Thank heavens my mother turned into our fairy godmother. She paid $12,000 to get our house out of foreclosure in exchange for my five-carat diamond ring. My mother also bought Luke and me a small house and put it in her trust. Our deal was that she would pay the mortgage until I could get back on my feet. Cinderella was back in rags, but at least she and her little prince were cared for and safe.

It took years for Luke and me to regain our balance after the divorce. My heart was broken, but my son was shattered. Through no fault of his own, at the age of 10, he lost everything that defined security for a child: home, family permanence, financial safety, friends, school, and the prestige that went along with our lavish lifestyle. More precursors for addiction had walked into his life and dug into his tender heart.[1]

Two thousand five was a taxing year, and I looked forward to a relaxing summer. Luke's father was in federal prison for obstructing and impeding the administration of the IRS, leaving me alone to deal with all of life's peculiarities. Our sole provider, I secured an adjunct teaching position at Fayetteville State University. The faculty bathroom became the perfect place to cry between classes. Dealing with a hormonal teen is a contest unto itself under normal conditions. Yet normal had left us in the dust years ago. To say I was overwhelmed was an understatement.

By age 14, Luke turned into a hermit. He spent a great deal of time alone in his room playing video games. Luke complained of his tailbone hurting, but I assumed it was because he was glued to his chair. It wasn't until he showed me a large bump at the bottom of his spine that I began to take his complaint seriously and took him to a doctor.

Puberty swept over Luke in what seemed like one weekend. Little did I know that early puberty, also called precocious puberty, was

Chapter 2. The Little White Pill

another precursor to addiction. Puberty's gift to Luke was terrible cystic acne. A pilonidal cyst had formed at the base of his spine. Surgery was the only option, followed by two weeks of bed rest flat on his stomach … so much for a relaxing summer at the pool.

Luke's personality changed after the surgery. Suddenly he was happy, or so it seemed. A lovely nurse gave him a little white pill called Oxycontin for pain. That little white pill not only took away the pain of the surgery but it also took away his depression, heartache, and anger. From that moment on, it was on his radar but not on mine. Why should it be? Oxycodone was the new wonder drug. My son was finally healing, and that was all that mattered.

Hidden from the public was that Purdue Pharma had convinced the medical profession and the FDA that Oxycontin had only a 1 percent chance of addiction. Doctors began passing the drug out like candy.[2]

When Luke was 15, he had his wisdom teeth pulled—another round of Percocet, which was Tylenol and Oxycodone. Sprained thumb—Oxy. Thumb surgery—Oxy. A sizeable wooden sliver in his

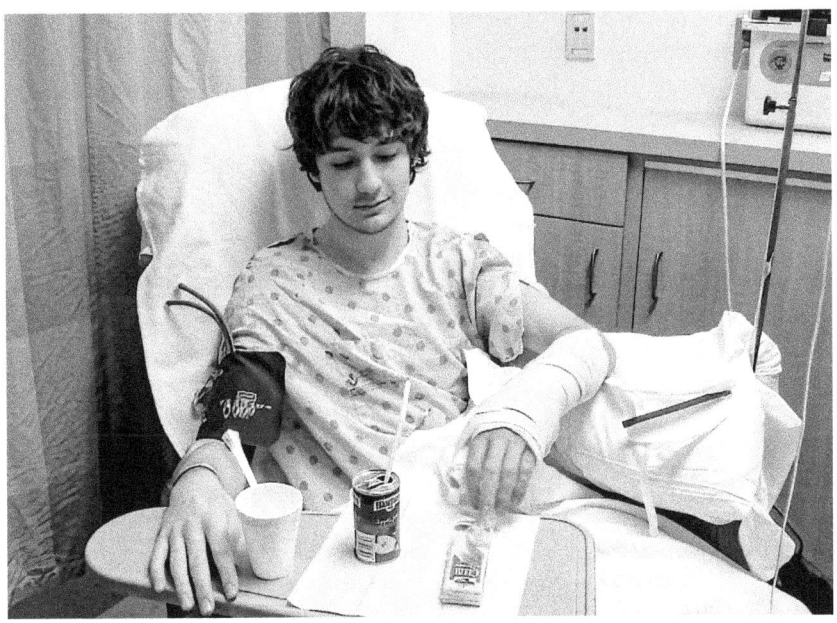

Luke, age 14, thumb surgery. Oxy round two.

foot when he was 16—Oxy. I was there. I saw it. I trusted the doctors and this new miracle pain pill. Doctors were prescribing it with little to no understanding that Purdue had intentionally skewed the graphs leading them to think it was not addictive. But Oxycodone is addictive, dangerously addictive, and it was taking control of my son.

Luke had no trouble feigning a physical problem to get what he wanted. When he couldn't obtain any Percocet, he drank to keep from detoxing. Little did I know that the drugs altered Luke's developing brain, making it harder for him to make his own "feel good" chemicals like serotonin and dopamine. He was hiding his drug dependency like a pro.

When his medications ran out, he retreated to his room in despair. Beer cans, lots of them, started appearing under his bed. His moods became erratic. His behavior took a deviant turn. I was mortified but didn't know what to do. Every time I addressed his drinking, he raged at me.

Did I see my son's drug dependency developing? No. I trusted the doctors. Did I know he was substituting substances when I found a bong in his room? No. Just a passing phase, I thought. I could not see beyond my pain to see what was happening to my boy. I chalked it all up to a hard adolescence, hoping he'd grow out of it. He didn't.

Luke acted out and got into trouble at school and with the law. I pointed out Luke's beer drinking and prescription drug use to his dad, but Baxter vehemently denied a substance abuse problem. "Just boys being boys," he'd say.

I, on the other hand, was devastated and bewildered. I did not raise my son to be a delinquent—quite the opposite. As a pastor's daughter, I ensured he had a solid foundation in the church. His actions humiliated me, yet my love for him demanded I forgo my ego and seek professional help.

Not quite able to see the situation for what it was, I took Luke to a psychiatrist who diagnosed him as bipolar. At first, I denied the diagnosis but then quickly saw I could blame his detrimental actions on this mental disorder. What an easy excuse. Luke already had ADD, GAD, OCD, and Tourette's—all neurological conditions. Bipolar made sense and thus took the onus off me to face the real problem.

First came the prescription Depakote. No, that didn't work. Then

Chapter 2. The Little White Pill

the Seroquel. Then the lithium. Then the combinations of all of them. Nothing helped. As a matter of fact, they all made him act crazy, and his behavior worsened.

One night we went to the grocery store. Luke was in one of his manic modes, which, quite frankly, could be pretty entertaining. During his manic moments, his bubbly personality and quick wit intensified. It was not so delightful in public, however. While picking out some produce, Luke loudly broke into his own Broadway musical version of "I Love My Momma," complete with tap dancing. I froze. The whole store turned to view the extravaganza. I quickly tossed the veggies back in the bins and corralled him out the front door frantically, trying unsuccessfully to explain his condition to the cashiers.

"Did you take your medication, Luke?" I railed at him while dragging him out to the car.

"I did, I did, I did, I did! I took my pills, Momma!" Luke sang happily to the tune of "Sit Down You're Rockin' the Boat" from *Guys and Dolls*. I simply put my head on the steering wheel and cried.

Enough is enough! The psychiatrist didn't know what he was doing—he only knew his field, which was to prescribe meds. I fired him and took Luke to a psychologist. After a lengthy interview, he gave his opinion that Luke was not bipolar but a highly creative yet depressed young man who had become chemically dependent. By 17, Luke was caught in the web of drugs, using anything he could get his hands on to make his anxiety and pain disappear. I had no clue about the bio-neurological changes occurring in his brain. It is nearly impossible to "just say no" as the drug-dependent brain screams, "You stop, I die!"

No parent wants to admit their child has a drug dependency. My dreams for Luke were dissipating. *What will people think?* haunted my waking hours. My fears and lack of understanding clouded me from seeing the truth. Disgust, anger, and blame kept me steeped in shame. Yet the stark reality in front of me begged that I pay attention. I cried myself to sleep too many nights, making excuses. It crushed me to admit that my son was addicted to drugs, and yet I knew we'd both drown in denial if I didn't accept that fact.

Pride be dammed! I called Luke's grandparents, begging for help. They arrived the next day.

We had a consult with the medical doctor on staff at a mental health clinic, and he instructed us to taper off Luke's meds slowly. Weaning off all medications would be dangerous. Yet there was no detox unit at our local hospital. We could not take Luke to the ER unless he was in crisis.

Luke started to crash after tapering off the meds. I tucked him in bed, trying to remember the sweet face of my baby, his arms reaching out for his final snuggle of the night. My anguished son, wrenching in pain, was looking back at me instead, clinging to me for dear life. To see him suffer so terribly destroyed me. My heart was writhing in pain with each of his tremors and cries for help. After hours of heartbreaking agony, he finally drifted off to sleep in my arms. My tears mingled with his on the pillow.

Luke slept for more than 30 hours. He shook violently in his sleep, his sweat soaking the sheets. Someone was always at his bedside to monitor his breathing. When he woke up, he was groggy but calm, thrilled to see his grandparents. We went out for a late breakfast to reconnect and make plans for his recovery.

I spoke with Luke's new psychologist, who said, "There's this new drug called Suboxone. It could help Luke stay off narcotics."[3]

"What exactly is it?" I asked.

"It's an opioid antagonist that can curb Luke's cravings. He'll eventually need a step-down from Suboxone, like other, more dangerous opioids."

I reflected on his words, recalling Luke's struggle when fighting cravings, then said, "If you think it can help…. Can you write him a prescription?"

"Well, the problem is," he went on to say, "only a medical physician with an X-waiver can write one. The X-waiver requires eight hours of continuing education, and even then, the physicians who can prescribe it can only accept up to 10 patients."

Really? What sense does that make? I thought. *Why can so many medical professionals pass out narcotics without oversight, but only a handful of them are allowed to prescribe Suboxone, a drug that could turn off the cravings and help end addiction?* I began to get the first glimpse of what was truly happening between pharmaceutical companies, medical practitioners, and public policy, but I had no idea why.[4]

I went home and did as the psychologist suggested. I scoured the

Internet for doctors who could prescribe Suboxone. I found only three doctors in North Carolina and chose the closest one, 120 miles away.

Luke was more than willing to see this doctor as he was tired of failures in academics and his personal life. His confidence was at an all-time low. Luke had been attending Interlochen Arts Academy during his junior year of high school. Even though he was artistically successful, he was behind academically in his credit hours. He was not excelling enough to be invited back to school in September, another blow to his self-confidence.

We did find a physician to provide Luke with counseling and Suboxone. Over the next few months, Luke weaned off of Suboxone and began getting his life back. He promptly took the GRE and passed with high scores. He knew he was smart and wanted to go on to college. Luke also knew walking a path of sobriety would be the only way to attain his goals. At last, some light was breaking through the storm clouds.

*****

Meanwhile, I was busy with work on the tenure track at Fayetteville State University. I also taught an online class at Sandhills Community College and accepted a part-time position one day a week directing our church's children's worship arts program. I needed the extra income; the additional jobs provided more money for Luke and me. While Baxter was in prison, Luke's brother Worth was kind enough to pay the child support. It was an act of love that endeared him to Luke forever.

When spring term ended, I was exhausted and looking forward to spending a restful summer with Luke and my folks in Florida. The universe had other plans. When I arrived in late May, my mother told me she had just been diagnosed with breast cancer. Then, in June, Grandpa Joe started choking when he ate. What we thought was indigestion ended up being advanced esophageal cancer. Because of their age, they both refused chemo and radiation. They wanted to live out their days together without all the medical mess. We all took a deep breath and prepared for what was to come. I became the sole caregiver as no other children in the families stepped up to the plate. End-of-life care demands much more than a weekly phone call.

Luke was devastated. Grandpa was Luke's hero, and Grandma was his rock who fiercely fought to keep him out of harm's way. As uncertainty loomed over Luke's future like an ominous storm cloud, his grandmother's love continually spoiled him, attempting to remind him of brighter days. I never knew what Luke would bring home after visiting his grandmother—big toys like computers, a leather satchel, designer suits, and watches. All the gifts in the world couldn't fill the void Luke inherently felt. And me? I was on autopilot, numb to the world, just putting one foot in front of the other, hoping not to trip and fall into the hole I had dug for myself.

Our lives changed quickly when Grandpa Joe passed away in mid-January 2010. After 21 years of marriage, my mother was alone while dealing with her slow-growing cancer and declining stamina. I could not leave my work, however. Luke was the only one with flexibility, so we agreed that he would take care of Grandma in Florida until I could work out better arrangements for her.

Three weeks after Grandpa Joe passed away, the unthinkable happened.

It was hard to accept that Luke was moving to Florida. I dreaded living alone again, with only Katie, our Golden Retriever, as company. Yet, as much as I knew I would miss him, I knew it was in everyone's best interest. My schedule was grueling, teaching classes, working with the church youth music program, and directing plays in the evening. We'd never see each other anyway. My mom was now alone and needed her boy more than I did. She was still too independent to move in with me. I wanted him to stay with me until his 19th birthday on February 11, but I could tell from Mom's voice she needed him sooner. I would have to wait until spring break to see them both. So be it.

With loving reluctance, I helped Luke pack his old Range Rover on February 3. We met his dad that night for a pre-birthday celebration. Baxter had finally come to terms with the divorce and, in his way, was trying to come to terms with Luke's move.

My mother was beside herself with joyful anticipation. With Mom's blessing, Yarrow, Luke's first love and steady girlfriend, would join him in a few weeks. Much to my surprise, Mom had no problem with them sharing a bedroom. Was the woman who had given me hundreds of lectures on the evils of sex before marriage just tossing out her old rule book?

Chapter 2. The Little White Pill

Luke left late the following day; he would spend the night at a hotel midpoint. Returning to the road late the next morning, he headed to Naples, Florida. He set his GPS on the most direct route that did not include the interstate, which took him on a rural road through a small town called Arcadia. I was expecting a call from my mother any minute telling me of his safe arrival. Instead, at 4 p.m., I received a phone call from a stranger.

"Is this Susan Paschal?" a voice asked.

"Yes," I replied, feeling a sense of unknown dread.

"Your son has been in an accident. He gave me your number and wanted me to call you to tell you he loves you."

"What? Come again?" I replied, stunned. *Was this another one of Luke's dramas?* My initial response was that he was in a minor mishap and didn't want me to get mad, so he had someone else break the news.

"Can I talk to him?" I asked.

"We were just passersby when it happened. We've called an ambulance."

Oh, my Lord, no. This incident was no prank. No dramatic ploy.

"Is he OK?" I didn't have the courage to ask if he was alive.

"Someone will call you soon," the man said caringly as he ended the call.

Apparently, Luke had been run off the road by a passing car. He overcorrected and lost control. Only two hours away from Naples. Not wearing a seatbelt, he was ejected from the car's side window and slammed to the ground as the vehicle spiraled down the road. A passing paramedic also stopped right after the accident occurred. He took one look at Luke and immediately called for air medical transport.

"We've already called an ambulance," replied one of the spectators.

"He'll never make it. We need to get him to a trauma center ASAP. Luckily, it's only 30 miles away," the paramedic shouted, returning to his car and announcing, "I'll be right back. I live just a mile down the road. I'm going to get my emergency kit."

When he returned, Luke stopped breathing as blood poured from his nose and mouth. The ambulance was nowhere in sight. The paramedic quickly bagged Luke and used mild compressions since he could see Luke's chest had been crushed. The medical transport helicopter landed two minutes later and the trauma team took over. There were angels all over Luke that day.

Meanwhile, I relayed the information to Luke's father. Baxter quickly called the Florida Highway Patrol, who said, "Get here as fast as you can—things don't look hopeful."

How do we get from North Carolina to Florida fast? There were no more flights that day, so Baxter and I decided to make the 12-hour drive together. Baxter didn't tell me the extent of the injuries. All he said was, "Luke is hurt, and we need to get down there quickly."

I threw some things in a bag and waited for him to pick me up. I put all of my pain and anger toward Baxter from the divorce on hold. Our son was all that mattered.

Within an hour, we were on the road. Then, panic struck again. *What to do about Mom?* I couldn't just call and tell her. She was alone, probably cooking a big meal to welcome Luke, as he was due there any minute.

Luckily, I knew my mother's pastor and called to inform him of the situation. He quickly drove to my mother's house, broke the news, and took her to the hospital. The nurses allowed her five minutes with Luke as he was in critical condition. Undeterred, my mother sent the pastor home, telling him she would call a friend to get her later. With the calm of an angel, Mom settled herself at Luke's bedside in the ICU-ER and began singing hymns, stroking his bloodied hair, and whispering loving words of encouragement. The medical staff came in to do assessments around her. Finally, at midnight, the nurses asked her to leave.

"I think not," Mom replied, never looking up at them. She was not about to let him die on her watch.

*****

The 12-hour drive felt like an eternity. I sat frozen, counting every stripe on the interstate. Baxter occasionally called the hospital for an update. He wouldn't say much after he hung up except "He's in critical condition, Susan, but he's still with us."

My mantra became *Please, dear God, keep my baby alive. Please, dear God, keep my baby alive.* Reality hit me that Luke could die, and I retreated to my safe place. I went numb.

Day One

We arrived at the hospital at 5 a.m. I walked into his room to see my son on a ventilator doing his breathing for him. Tubes filled with blood ran down the sides of his bed as they drained his lungs. Eight different bags of drugs hung on the IV pole, pouring into his motionless body. A large gash ran along the left side of his face, barely missing his eye. Crude stitches held his face together. He was in critical condition with little chance of survival. The nurse on duty patted my hand and told me it might be best to say my goodbyes. *No way in hell!* I screamed to myself. He was still with me.

I simply took Luke's hand and told him, "Momma Bear is here. You're going to be OK, Bug."

"You are too, honey," whispered my mother behind me as she gathered her belongings. "I'll see you tonight."

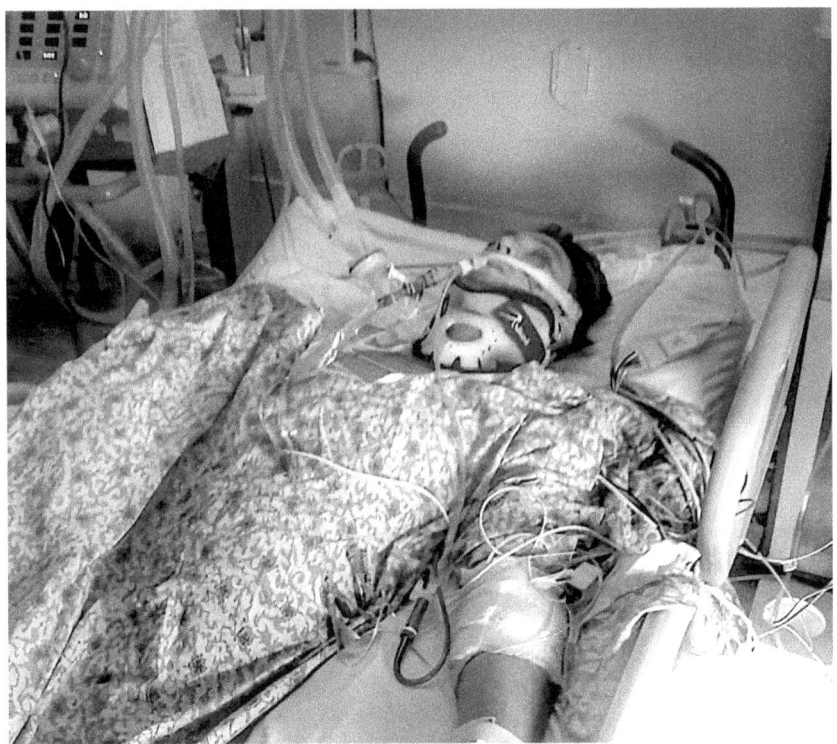

This is what life support looks like after a near-fatal car accident. Day One.

Day Two

Luke made it through the first 24 hours, but his condition was still critical. I remained hunkered down in my spot next to him, my eyes glued to the blinking monitors as he breathed in sync with the clangs of his ventilator, fighting for his life. Even though he was in a deep drug-induced coma, I kept stroking his hair, reassuring him everything would be OK.

The attending physician came in around 10:00 a.m. She said, "Luke's injuries are extensive. His midsection is crushed. He suffered lacerations to his face. Fortunately, no brain swelling, neck fractures, or neurological problems have been detected."

Thank God! I prayed silently as she continued.

She said, "Unfortunately, Luke's back is severely broken in multiple places, leaving his legs paralyzed. We can't schedule surgery until his vital signs stabilize."

The medical staff lightened Luke's coma drugs at noon, and he squeezed my hand. I finally drew my first full breath since receiving the phone call. Luke immediately showed signs of intense pain and was placed back in a deep coma.

The nurse said, "He's doing better, but pneumonia and infection are always threats when someone is intubated."

Fear gripped me again. I stared at all the ports, drains, and tubes attached to his mangled body and asked, "When can you schedule surgery to fix Luke's T-6 burst fracture?"

"When we think he has a chance of survival, ma'am. Twenty-four hours is good. Forty-eight is even better. If he makes it to 72, he may have a fighting chance," she replied cautiously.

Day Three

As we feared, pneumonia was setting in, and Luke's fever and pulse escalated—as did my blood pressure. Yet he was fighting and getting stronger.

The doctors, nurses, and therapists assigned to Luke's case usually gathered around 10:00 a.m. Much of the medical jargon was beyond my understanding, such as "mainline subclavian port and an IVC filter for blood clots." I deferred to Baxter, who handled the paperwork. As a chiropractic physician, he understood the medicalese.

The doctors brought Luke out of the coma to test his leg responses. He wiggled his toes on his right foot! What a gift! The entire room broke out in cheers. Luke also weakly opened his eyes, squeezed my hand, and tried to move his lips around the tube like he was asking for a kiss—a request I was more than happy to oblige.

Six p.m. came too soon, and we had to leave him. Our next task was to set up a base camp at Mom's. Luke's recovery would take weeks at the hospital and many more months at home. Thankfully, my niece Jenni had flown in the night before. She immediately took on the job as my functioning brain, warm headrest, and gracious assistant. Yarrow, Luke's girlfriend, arrived later in the day. Even though we were divorced, Baxter and I loved our son and clung to each other as he clung to life.

Forty-eight hours down. Twenty-four more to go to reach the safe zone.

Day Four

I kissed my mother goodbye at 5:45 a.m., and then Baxter, Jenni, Yarrow, and I drove to the hospital to visit Luke. The news when we arrived was not promising. Luke's blood pressure had dipped dangerously low during the night, and six units of blood and medications were used to bring him back into the safe zone.

By 2:00 p.m., Luke had become unresponsive. The medical team administered a CAT scan and found a small part of his left lung collapsing, so they installed a drain, but at least the pneumonia was abating.

The nurses brought Luke to his room and took him off the Propofol, the coma medication. Yarrow's damp, smiling eyes were the first to greet him when he woke. I held her upright as she almost fainted, seeing him injured and incapacitated for the first time. Luke could barely communicate, but her presence was indeed the best medicine as they held each other's hands.

Luke made it to the 72-hour mark.

Day Five

Luke's regular nurse, Patty, caught me panicking whenever one of Luke's monitors changed beep patterns. She tried to calm me but to no avail. I was sure we were losing him and no one was responding.

Finally, Patty took me by the shoulders and said, "Susan, you have absolutely no idea what information these monitors give us. I do. They give trends. Not absolutes. Listen, if you see me afraid, then you can be afraid." She demonstrated this with a big, scary frown and continued, "If you see I am not afraid," she said, giving me a big, happy smile, "then everything is good. Let's practice."

We did. Big, happy smiles—big, scary frowns.

"Got it?" she asked.

"Got it!" I replied, sharing a much-needed laugh with her.

From that moment on, I'd look for her smiling face when I entered the room and then begin to breathe on my own.

On day five, I walked into Luke's room early in the morning, and Patty quickly turned her face away from me. She was not smiling. Then I noticed the room was abuzz with medical staff and saw scores of empty bags of blood dangling from the IV pole. The chief surgeon ran into the room and started asking questions, all foreign medical talk to me.

"Take him to surgery," barked the doctor.

I understand that!

"When?" the staff replied.

"STAT!"

The staff moved instantly with precision as they rushed Luke's bed and the attached paraphernalia out the door. Patty also left, leaving me alone with Yarrow. We held on to each other and made our way down to the waiting room. Jenni fetched Baxter to meet us there.

While we were in the waiting room, we found out Luke had flatlined during the night. He was bleeding out. A code blue was called. Patty sat on his chest doing compressions as the staff went through 20 units of blood trying to keep him alive. They had only three units of his blood type left before they would be forced to let Luke die. He was stabilized only minutes before I entered his room. Hearing about the events made me cave in terror and gratitude.

Chapter 2. The Little White Pill

Five hours later, Luke was out of surgery. All went well, considering he had a chest full of broken ribs, a collapsed lung, a crushed sternum, facial wounds, a lacerated liver, a bruised pancreas, and a perforated intestine. The intestine was down to the final membrane. If that membrane had been severed, he would have died from sepsis. His spleen had ruptured, causing the bleed out, and was removed. Miracles kept abounding. We needed them to keep coming. The surgeon had not even started to think about repairing his broken back.

Day Six

I walked into Luke's room early in the morning to find his hands in mitts and nurse Patty's hands on her hips. She smiled at me—a big smile. *Oh, thank God.*

"Luke was a naughty boy last night. He pulled out his chest tubes. Now we must bind him up so he keeps his little piddies off his medicine port," Patty said in a loving but chiding voice. "It was a good thing he didn't need them anymore."

"Seriously, son?"

Luke just grinned. I instantly noticed Luke breathing independently without the ventilator for the first time. I tried to breathe too as Luke gave me a weak smile and said, "Hi, Momma."

Hearing my son's voice for the first time since the accident brought tears to my eyes. I smiled warmly, resisting the urge to hug him and smother him with kisses. "Hi, Bug," I replied softly.

"He's got quite a story to tell you, Mom," Patty teased as she picked up her chart. She and Jenni left the room to give me a moment with Luke. I smothered him with my usual light hugs and fairy kisses, trying hard not to jiggle the bed.

"We almost lost you, son…"

"I know, Momma," he whispered. After a long pause, he said, "It's really beautiful over there."

"Over where, son?" I saw nothing beautiful outside his window.

"I was on the other side with Grandpa."

I paused for a long time, not knowing how to respond. Finally, I said, "Oh … really?"

Luke went on fervently. "We talked for a long time. It was so beautiful. I didn't hurt anymore. There were friendly beings of light who were warm and welcoming. I saw Jesus, too, I think. I couldn't see his face, but it felt like it could be him. So kind … accepting. Big Dude…"

"What?" I gasped quietly.

"The voice told me I had more do to. I wasn't ready to cross over but didn't have to return because I was so badly hurt. It said recovery would be very tough. I was given a choice and had to think hard about it. But oh, those loving lights, towering green trees. Beautiful music, angels singing. Oh, the music, Mom … the music … no pain…" Luke's voice trailed off.

I took a long, deep breath.

"What made you choose to come back, honey?" I asked through my tears.

"You…" he whispered with a tired smile as he fell back to sleep.

*****

When we arrived at the hospital the next day, Luke was in stable condition. It was also Luke's 19th birthday, but he was too out of it to celebrate. His birthday cake was administered through a feeding tube. His spirits seemed high, however, after seeing the birthday cards sent from people from our church. The nurses made a surprise display for him, complete with balloons.

His best birthday present came from the chief doctor who announced, "Chances are good Luke is going to pull through."

The present I received was that Luke could move both legs again, so the surgeon scheduled the back surgery for the following day.

It was a grand day, but my heart was troubled. As I left Luke's room that night, out of the corner of my eye, I zeroed in on the multiple bags of drugs hanging from his bed. Ketamine, fentanyl, morphine, to name only three of the many pouring into his body, high dosages that would continue for weeks to come. Fear chilled me to my bones. I knew we would fight a bigger demon down the road, one that would not heal with time.

Week Two

Luke's back surgery was long and complicated. Baxter and I waited with the girls in the family area. After three hours, the doctor came to give us the news.

"Dr. and Mrs. Paschal, your son did just fine," the surgeon announced.

I smiled in relief but inwardly grimaced at my old title. It was not the time to correct others about our marital status.

The surgeon explained, "The multiple spinal fractures will heal on their own, but his T-6 vertebra is crushed. To fix it, I did a procedure called vertebroplasty. We injected a glue-type substance into the body of the vertebra. Two titanium rods and eight screws were placed along the spine for further stabilization. Unfortunately, Luke will forever have a limited range of motion, but the rods have made his back stronger than it was before. He'll be back in his room within the hour."

We thanked the doctor, and I went to the chapel to gather my thoughts. *How lucky we are*, I thought repeatedly. The eight-inch scar on Luke's back and the 18-inch scar down his abdomen would heal in time. Plastic surgery could fix his face after a year. Luke lost two inches of his height. He would no longer be 6'1 because the surgery condensed his spine and left him with a slight hunch. It was a small price to pay.

Week Three—Step Down

We were happy when the hospital staff gave orders for Luke's discharge from the ICU and transferred him to the fifth floor. Trepidation set in when there was no longer a private room with his wonderful nurse Patty and the reassurance of the ICU's immediate care response.

During his transfer, the head surgeon said his goodbyes to Luke and to us and told Luke, "If anyone ever asks you if you've won the lottery, Luke, you can truthfully say yes."

I could tell the doctor meant what he said, and I felt a wave of gratitude for the gift of Luke's life. Luke was a living miracle. The rest of us were a shaking mess.

*****

Recovery would be a long haul. Luke would stay in the hospital for a few more weeks while weaning off the high dosage of morphine and switching to Oxycontin to help him manage his pain. We were told when Luke was strong enough to leave the hospital, he would have to stay in a stable environment and couldn't travel by plane or take a long car ride for months.

It was clear that Luke would need hourly care and a supportive place to heal his damaged body. The broken bones would heal faster than all the damaged soft tissue, not to mention the mental trauma of the accident. My mother and I decided it would be best for Luke to stay with her in Florida while Baxter and I had to return to North Carolina for work. Yarrow, Luke's girlfriend, volunteered to stay in Naples to care for Luke and Grandma. What an angel! As much as I hated to admit it, it was for the best as I could not care for him properly at home with my three-job schedule.

The thought of leaving my son was excruciating. Baxter and I worked out a parental tag team schedule, traveling back and forth from North Carolina to visit Luke at Grandma's in Florida for the next few weeks. I had almost lost my boy and was still struggling to catch my breath.

The night before I left, Luke consoled me more than I reassured him. We held hands and made wild plans for what we would do when he got better, then quietly sang our song, "Over the Rainbow / Wonderful World," the Israel Kamakawiwo'ole version, as he drifted off to sleep.

I found my mother awake in her office when I returned from the hospital. My heart broke for her too. She was 86, dealing with her cancer diagnosis, had just lost her second husband, and had almost seen her cherished grandson die before her. Yet there she was, stoic and resilient like the Rock of Gibraltar.

"How do you stay so strong, Momma?" I asked, sinking into the side chair.

She just patted her Bible and smiled. "My faith. I did not intend to lose Luke, but I knew I would be close behind if I did, and he would be the first to greet me at heaven's gate. That alone gave me peace."

She ignored the *What about me?* look on my face.

"Thank you for loving us both so much, Momma. I don't know

what I would have done without you all these years," I admitted as the tears started to flow.

She nodded as she also wiped away a tear. "If not for your family, then for who, honey? Don't forget, I was also carrying him when I was carrying you."

I had never thought about that. "Yes, I guess you did."

However, it was time to pack, as Baxter and I had a long drive ahead of us back to North Carolina first thing in the morning. Thankfully our trip home was much less stressful than the drive down.

*****

My anxiety mounted as the weeks went on. I felt helpless being 700 miles away from Luke. As expected, I called my mother and Yarrow multiple times a day. Their updates from Luke's aftercare nurses were encouraging. Mom and Yarrow told me Luke was progressing, walking a few steps each day. They also said his pain was escalating, which concerned me but didn't seem to concern them.

My first lesson in pain management was beginning. The doctors called what Luke was experiencing "breakthrough pain," a term that Purdue Pharma, the manufacturer of Oxycontin, pushed for doctors to accept and share with patients like Luke. Doctors informed me that "not treat[ing] pain could be a cause for malpractice. The medical community is now diagnosing pain as the fifth vital sign."[5]

Only a few physicians understood the newly coined term "breakthrough pain." Dr. Alfred Clavel, Jr., concisely wrote about it in his Health Partners blog "5 Ways Opioids and Their Negative Side Effects Make Your Pain Worse." "Opioids provided relief by blocking pain; however, the body reacted by increasing the number of receptors to get the pain signal through to the brain again. So, when the drug wore off, a person experienced more pain. If they continued to take opioids, the pills became less and less effective. As tolerance increased, a patient needed more and more medication to get pain relief."[6]

To overcome Luke's breakthrough pain, doctors upped his dosage to 160 mg per day of Oxycontin, which seemed high, and his dosage increased every time I called for an update. Doctors typically prescribe less than half that for bone recovery patients and between 200 and 600 mg daily for late-stage cancer patients. More than that, one risked overdose from respiratory failure.

The reports from Florida regarding Luke's dosages became more and more concerning because I understood Luke's history with addiction. Finally, I couldn't wait in North Carolina any longer. *To hell with it*, I thought as I packed my bags for Florida. My son needs me, and I will be there for him. Thankfully my colleagues picked up my classes, allowing me the privilege of going to him.

Unbeknownst to me, our first dance with the devil was just beginning.

Chapter 3

The Price Tag

"Everything has a price. The price, however, isn't always money."—Ahmed Mostafa

Off I went down I-95 to Florida, filling the 12-hour drive with music and gratitude, trying to forget the terror of the trip immediately after Luke's accident. I was still in a state of shock. At least, that is what we called it in those days. The term PTSD was reserved for service members traumatized in combat, for the most part, or victims of assault. My son survived, yet I was still quaking, repeating the mantra *He almost died, he almost died, my baby almost died.*

Visiting hours were long over when I drove past the hospital in Fort Myers. A tear rolled down my cheek as I blew Luke a kiss goodnight as I sped by. One more cup of coffee. One more time listening to *Les Mis*. One more hour to Mom's and I could sleep.

Of course, Mom was up waiting for me when I walked in the door. She simply smiled, put down her Bible, and kissed me goodnight. The woman seemed cool as a cucumber on the outside, but I knew she had been up and fervently praying all evening, making little bargains with the angels. Yarrow tippy-toed in to give me a sleepy hug and kiss.

Looking around, I saw Grandma's house had been totally transformed. Her office was now in Joe's old room. Luke and Yarrow had a spacious, fully furnished room in the back with their private bathroom: new sheets, new furniture, new everything. Mom's old office was now a guest/rehab room complete with two different walkers, a wheelchair, a cane, and hand weights. I struggled to find a place for my luggage as I maneuvered to the bed. The girls had set up camp for the long haul of recovery. Maybe I was not as needed as I thought. With a sigh, I fell asleep exhausted but at peace, knowing I'd see my son the next day.

I was awake before dawn to review my checklist. Life had been a blur since the accident, and even I could tell my actions had become robotic.

We knew we had to wait for the hospital's morning call before we could get Luke. At noon he was cleared to go. Checkout time was 1:00. Off we went in two cars with Grandma in the lead.

Before seeing Luke, we were escorted into a small room to talk to the aftercare coordinator. She went through the litany of instructions and scripts to be filled. It was sobering to hear that Luke was out of the woods but far from being healed. His excellent accomplishment yesterday was walking to the nurses' station without getting out of breath. One lung was 100 percent, but the other was still slightly collapsed with fluid.

"You're letting him out of the hospital like this?" I gasped.

"This is a trauma center, ma'am; Luke is not in crisis anymore and…"

"His insurance ran out, I bet," I blurted out. Where was my filter when I needed it?

She did not answer, but her expression said it all. She continued, "Luke's white blood cell counts are slowly dropping—around 20,000 yesterday with slow drops each day. The doctors are confident Luke will be OK once he starts moving around. He is getting his stomach staples taken out now in his room. Next week you are to schedule an appointment to remove his back staples." Yarrow was scribbling away, taking copious notes.

How could I have possibly thought this was going to be easy? Reality hit. Dang my Pollyanna attitude! Luke would not be able to take care of himself for several months. He could not even begin to dress, and he could not perform even the simplest of tasks we all take for granted, like tying our shoes, going to the bathroom, and taking a shower alone.

"Everything is ready at home. We will be fine. I will be his primary caretaker, and Yarrow will help," Mom announced.

Oh, Ma, how could you have agreed to care for him at home when you can barely make it down the block without your walker? I barely managed to keep that thought to myself. *Then again, Susan, how could you just sit back and agree? Well, what was I supposed to do? What are my options? I have none.* This messy internal dialogue flew through my

Chapter 3. The Price Tag

head while my face just smiled and my head nodded in passive agreement while I signed all the necessary paperwork.

Before the nurse left, I asked her about the prescriptions that needed refilling.

"I understand the scripts to help with blood clots and white cell counts, but you only have a two-week script of Oxycontin for Luke. These are for 40 mg two times a day, which is much less than he takes now." I had been keeping track as this was not our first dance with narcotics.

"That's all he needs," the nurse replied.

"Excuse me? Whoa! Last week I told the nursing staff that Luke had been mildly dependent on narcotics before his accident and that he will need to be tapered off slowly from his current dose and then moved to Suboxone," I frantically reminded her.

"Oh, I'm sorry, but that was not in the notes." She looked clueless.

"Can you call the doctor, please?" I pleaded. "I cannot leave this hospital with this script. He will start to detox, which will be devastating in the condition he is in."

"I'm sorry, ma'am, I'll check, but this is all the doctors prescribed. Besides, no one here can write a script for Suboxone. We don't have a qualified doctor on staff. You'll have to find a primary care physician or pain management doctor to help you." Off she went, never to be seen or heard from again. Panic started settling in.

*****

Damn, I was in trouble, and I knew it. The pain meds they had given us might get Luke through four to five days at most. My mind was plotting. Game plan: As soon as I got to Mom's, I would make a few phone calls and find a doctor who understood Luke's unique situation. First things first, however. We had to get this broken boy home and in bed.

"Momma! You're back!" Luke called to me weakly as he was wheeled into the lobby. My heart jumped with joy, and I tried not to hurt him with a hug. Tears were running down both our faces. Finally, I could take a deep breath.

Grandma was already waiting for Luke in her car with pillows in the front seat. We carefully loaded him in and watched her drive off.

She had her boy back, and so did I. Yarrow and I packed all his belongings and medical equipment in our car and followed close behind.

After getting Luke settled in, I called Dr. Rebecca Estes for advice. Rebecca was a dear friend who had known Luke as a child. We met in our church choir and quickly became close friends as she had also survived a devastating divorce. She was also one of the few anesthesiologists who had taken the time to take a substance abuse rotation as part of her medical training.

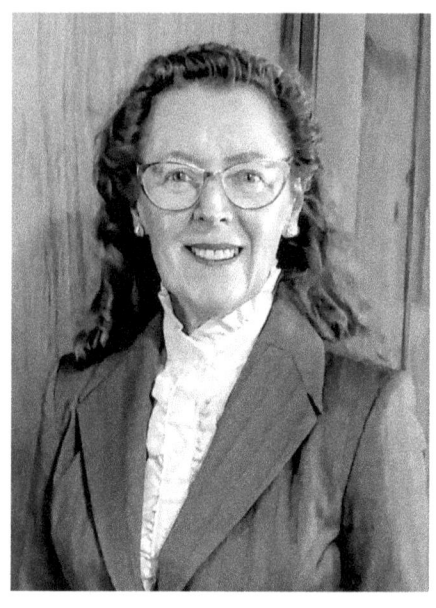

My dear friend and emotional life support, Dr. Rebecca Estes.

While searching for my phone and then for her number, I remembered those horrific days of drug misuse. Luke addicted? No. He just needed Percocet or he got nasty and sick. It was a dependency, not an addiction, right? A few times, the nurses were actually more concerned about the amount of Tylenol he was taking than the Oxycodone. Why should I be concerned if they were not? Addicts, after all, are junkies who stick needles in their arms and live in boxes on skid row. That was not my son. He was not a drug addict. Yet the questions remained. *Why could no one help us navigate our way out of these drugs?*

Thank heavens Rebecca had a few minutes to talk between her surgeries.

"Susan, I am so glad Luke survived. We were all praying—he's such a fine young man," she said with a deep sigh.

I quickly explained our situation and asked if she could take over Luke's medications. Her response surprised me.

"Oh, sweetie, I'm sorry I can't help you. Luke is in Florida. My license does not permit me to treat patients with narcotics out of state."

Damnit! "How about Suboxone? He was on it before. Can you send us some, just in case?" I pleaded in desperation.

Rebecca went on cautiously. She knew I was close to the edge. "No. I don't have a license to practice medicine in Florida. No drugs. Nothing. Suboxone is a controlled substance [CIII], too, because it contains buprenorphine—which is considered a narcotic. Susan, I am so sorry, but the law ties my hands. Besides, I am not his doctor, and neither one of us knows Luke's medical needs. You can't guess this out, as his mother."

"I understand. I didn't know I was asking you to do something illegal, Rebecca. I am so sorry," I muttered.

She paused, then continued. "I know you didn't, my friend. Listen, I need to warn you; some states are really cracking down on doctors prescribing narcotics right now. Florida is one of them. If a person illegally possesses more than 30 Oxycodone pills, they get charged with 'trafficking in Oxycodone,' an offense that carries a mandatory 15-year prison sentence."

"Mandatory? Seriously?" *Who would be stupid enough to do that?* I thought? Oh, silly me.

"Seriously, by law, they cannot make any exceptions," she warned. "You might even have to search for a doctor because many want nothing to do with narcotics anymore. They are abandoning their patients right and left."

"But he needs them, Rebecca. He's in a great deal of pain still. He's not faking it." I was starting to panic.

"Yes, I'm sure he needs it, but watch how much he is taking," she cautioned.

"I think he's up to 200 mg daily," I replied, scanning my broken memory banks.

"OK. What is happening, Susan, is that he has developed tolerance.[1] He has a high tolerance, like his father, most likely. His bones and internal injuries are healing, but his pain flares when the drug wears off, so he needs more of the same drug to get the same relief. It's a nasty cycle. And it's not his fault. It's how the drug makers intentionally designed it. Please remember that fact."

"Really?" I was trying to take it all in.

"Yes, people blame themselves for not being strong enough just to quit when in reality their brains can't function without it right away, causing them excruciating physical and mental pain."

"Detox." I remembered the painful process Luke had experienced before the accident.

"Yes. When you get back home, I'll explain more, but for now, you've got to get Luke the right care. He is probably using the drug to deaden his emotional pain too. He's done that before. You will need to address this issue immediately, as he has been through a traumatic ordeal, both physically and mentally. He needs a good therapist and an addictionologist, or at least a decent psychiatrist who truly understands addiction as a disease and not just a mental health issue, and then a treatment center when he is strong enough."

"A treatment center won't take him now?" I asked in disbelief.

"No. Oh no. Rehabs don't deal with anyone with Luke's type of injuries that require he still be on medication. And he still needs medical rehab—drug treatment centers are not designed for that kind of advanced care."

This news was unexpected. "You're telling me we have fallen between the cracks."

"Yes. Unfortunately, you have. An option is to admit Luke to a psychiatric hospital—but then he'd have to be tagged with a mental health disorder to be treated. Personally, I am not sure anyone there would know how to deal with his specific needs right now."

My mind was again racing. "Where can I find an addictionologist?"

"California, probably. There are none around here, and probably none in Florida. I took a medical addiction rotation at a treatment center because I had friends suffering and wanted to understand the disease better. Plus, I knew some anesthesia drugs could cause a trigger response. I'm afraid they don't teach addiction in medical school for more than a day, and there are just a handful of addiction fellowships in the country,"[2] she said sadly.

My heart sank, yet I kept pleading. "My son was almost killed in a car accident. Doctors saved him in part by issuing powerful, pain-relieving drugs. These same drugs, however, could damage his brain permanently if not administered properly. There are tens of thousands of people facing this same dilemma, yet only a handful of doctors in the country think it is a problem that deserves medical attention?"

"Pretty much," Rebecca replied.

"You can't help us at all?" I whimpered.

"No, honey, I'm sorry," Rebecca said apologetically. "When you get a doctor, call me. I'll be happy to talk to him about Luke's history as an observer. If he agrees, it will help me explain things better as they directly relate to Luke's situation. Hang in there, Susan. I'll see you when you get back."

I hung up the phone with dread in my heart and a looming task in front of me.

*****

Luke had taken some Oxycodone before he left the hospital, but he was in excruciating pain now due to the car ride up to this point. I gave him the amount he asked for, about three days' worth, counting on the fact that I'd be able to get a good doctor in the morning. Oh, how wrong I was—how naively and stupidly wrong.

The household was still sleeping when I woke up. Still in my pajamas, I started searching and making calls.

"Insurance, please?" the receptionist asked pleasantly.

"BCBS of NC," I proudly announced as I knew it had good coverage.

Her tone suddenly changed. "I'm sorry, that is out of network. Besides, we no longer take patients needing narcotics." Click.

Even though Rebecca had warned me this might happen, I was dumbfounded. What was the problem with narcotics? They were doctors. Drugs were medicine. I understood insurance snafus, but my son's life was at stake, for God's sake.

One doctor's office after another denied my requests.

Dear God, help! What was I supposed to do? My usual polite demeanor was not going to work in this situation. I was getting desperate.

When the last clinic on my list gave me the same reply, I sobbed, "Dear God, please help me. I am desperate. My son could die if someone doesn't help us! I cannot drive him back to North Carolina—it could kill him. I swear it's good insurance. The hospital just accepted payment for his hospital bill of $364,000!" I cried through the phone. "I'll give you a credit card to secure the payment!"

Thankfully the nurse recognized the desperation in my voice. She ditched the protocol and scheduled us with the pain management specialist for Tuesday. We had enough meds left to keep Luke comfortable until then. My mother gave me her credit card, which had a high limit, as mine did not.

"Thank you, God," I whispered as I sat at the table and wept into my cold coffee.

It had been five weeks since the accident. Luke was now down 50 pounds. He could barely walk from his bed to the bathroom, even with help. He was slurring his speech and hunched over, even in his brace. Every night he cried out in fear as he relived the crash in his dreams.

The next day it took us almost two hours to get Luke ready to see his new pain management doctor, who was thankfully 10 minutes from Mom's house.

Luke wanted to go in and see the doctor alone, however, and because he was 19 and thus an adult, I had no choice but to honor his wishes.

Luke looked greatly relieved as he came out in his wheelchair, script in hand. The nurse instructed him, "You have two weeks of 80 mg of Oxycodone that you must take three to four times daily. We'll reevaluate the amount at the next appointment. Do not hesitate to call if you start experiencing breakthrough pain."

Finally, I thought, we had someone who understood Luke's dependency. I was ignorantly confident the doctor could help him stay out of pain while slowly weaning him off the medication. Again, my naivete reared her ugly head. I did not know that the narcotics rules had drastically changed in the past five years. They were not in favor of the patient.

*****

We trust our doctors and the medical community to act in our best interest. After all, upon graduation from medical school, all doctors take the Hippocratic oath, which, in short, is a sworn agreement, a promise to share knowledge, to help the ill and not cause harm, and to never give a deadly drug or assist another to use one.[3]

Pharmaceutical companies, on the other hand, take no such oath. Most act responsibly, but Purdue Pharma did not. The Sackler family, who owned and operated Purdue, had created a powerful opioid painkiller called Oxycontin, an addictive narcotic once meant for acute end-of-life pain. Then, they intentionally marketed it as 1 percent addictive due to its time-release formula, claiming it could be used for mild to moderate pain. In short, Purdue knew Oxycontin was addictive and yet manipulated data, lied to the medical community, and then persuaded the FDA to adjust its labeling to make a profit. Billions of dollars in profit. By 2007, Purdue had gotten caught and been fined and some executives had been sentenced. Word was slow getting out to the public. Purdue was still cranking out the drug at record levels.[4]

Whereas Luke and I were blind to Purdue's selfish and irresponsible acts, law enforcement and the DEA were not. The NIH website reported that more than 44 percent of all drug-related fatalities that year were due to narcotics, the same kind that was about to turn our lives into a living hell.[5]

Policy change was in order, but the medical community did not know how to proceed. Doctors adopted one of three distinct types of ideologies regarding opioid addiction treatment.

The first followed the guidelines of the American Pain Foundation, of which Dr. Russell K. Portenoy was a director. The "King of Pain," the medical community called him. He urged tackling what was called an epidemic of "untreated pain." The doctors who took this approach believed it was inhumane not to treat a patient's discomfort. Many physicians feared being sued by their patients for undertreating them, resulting in people being dosed into addiction or death. Our current physician fell into this category.

The second approach, by far the most popular, was to crack down on prescribing narcotics and thus reduce the risk of doctors being sued for unintentional overdoses and/or getting sanctioned by state medical boards. Consequently, doctors were proud of themselves for not creating more addicts but gave no thought to the needs of those in their care who were already dependent on the drugs they initially prescribed. Physicians in this category simply cut their patients loose, essentially forcing them to buy their medication from "pill mills" or resort to alternatives like heroin off the streets.

The third approach was espoused by a small but significant group of doctors who realized that writing narcotics prescriptions was lucrative. One could safely call them licensed drug dealers. They remained well hidden, yet every addicted individual knew where to find them.

Unfortunately, our journey would lead us to all three types of pain management doctors. We could only move forward with what we knew.

*****

Besides spending quality time with Luke, I spent my spring break setting up aftercare appointments to leave me feeling secure or as secure as possible under the circumstances.

It was good to see Luke making progress while I was there. He was slowly able to put on his brace, shower by himself, and scoot around the house with a walker. His appetite was coming back, and he looked to be gaining weight. Other than the disfiguring scar on his face, I was starting to recognize my son again. I promised him we would get his scar fixed when the time came. He was worried about his face more than anything.

Meanwhile, my mother was busy finding good counselors to help Luke deal with the trauma of being tied down with a machine breathing for him. Luke was still having dreams of the accident that left him traumatized. At night I could hear him cry out, reliving each roll of the car before it spat him out on the pavement. The Xanax his doctor prescribed did little to calm his terrors and just zoned him out.

The day before I left to return to North Carolina, we took Luke to the hospital for his last aftercare check-ups. First, we saw the internist for blood work monitoring. Trends were looking better. The next stop was to see the physical therapist to enhance Luke's back's range of motion. It was a painful process. Our last visit was for the neurosurgeon to check Luke's back apparatus and his Tourette's as the jerks hurt his broken ribs and back.

The doctor checked Luke out and was pleased with the healing of all his broken bones. Yarrow took him to the car while we finished talking to the doctor and collecting the prescriptions. Luke was too exhausted to take in any more information.

My mother insisted on being involved in Luke's aftercare because he would be living with her and because she firmly believed in natural healing methods above pharmaceuticals.

Chapter 3. The Price Tag

"I will be taking over the medications," my mother announced, pointing out her name on the HIPPA form that Luke had signed.

I just shrugged and stepped aside.

"What is this one for?" my mother demanded.

"Muscle relaxers for Tourette's," the doctor calmly replied.

"And this one?"

"Omega 3. Luke needs it to support his bones and brain function."

Before I could intervene, my mother thrust the script back in the doctor's hand and barked in her professorial tone, "We don't need this Omega. We have our own."

A bit irritated, the doctor thrust the script back at her. "Lady, you can't buy this Omega off the shelf. It is pharmaceutical grade. The rest is junk. Trust me."

"We. Take. Shaklee," she retorted, pushing the script back at him once again.

I hung my head in embarrassment at her persistence but said nothing. My mother had partnered with Shaklee, a reputable nutraceutical company, for decades and believed in their products' efficacy almost as much as she believed in Jesus. Thankfully the doctor was aware of the company's stellar reputation and kept his script.

"That is an excellent brand, ma'am. Just make sure Luke takes the prescribed amount per day," he said with a sigh.

Mom looked at me with her famous *I told you so* glare as I wrote down the instructions. She was rather pleased with herself and backed off graciously. I looked on apologetically.

The neurosurgeon then went on with some other news that was difficult to hear.

"Luke's back was badly broken, as you well know. It is a miracle he is not paralyzed. The small fractures in his lumbar region will heal in time, but the spinal fusion at the T-6 burst fracture may be problematic in years to come."

He took out some X-rays to better show that the tabs on the end of the vertebrae were smaller than average. Because of that, he had to create a small bend in Luke's upper back when he attached the bone with rods and screws, thus causing Luke to lose two inches in height.

OK, we can deal with that one, I thought to myself, not understanding the full implication of the doctor's warning.

The doctor continued. "I'm pretty certain in the years to come, his apparatus will cause problems and need addressing."

"Another surgery?" I asked in disbelief.

"Most likely. But hopefully, by then, we will have new techniques to keep Luke mobile. Good luck," the doctor said in closing.

"Thank you, doctor." My heart sank as he walked away. I assumed Luke was fixed forever. After careful consideration, I thought it best not to share that information with Luke now. I didn't want him to start worrying about something that "might" happen. We had enough on our plate with what "had" happened.

We ended my visit to Naples with a nice dinner, followed by Yarrow and I packing up the car. She needed a break and was going back to North Carolina with me to audition at a neighboring university. I tucked everyone in that night with a promise of better days ahead and nabbed a few hours of sleep before Yarrow and I snuck out at dawn. I drove for 12 hours, lost in my fears, while Yarrow slept. *Would this pit in my stomach ever go away?*

Even though my mother sincerely appreciated Yarrow and me being there, she was happy to get us out of the house and have Luke to herself. I, however, was not so sure it was a good idea to leave a 5-foot-2 cancer-ridden 85-year-old woman to care for an injured, heavily-medicated 19-year-old man-child. Don't get me wrong, my mother was still as sharp as a tack, with North Dakota grit that could take on the most formidable opponent. Other than her slow-growing cancer, which she denied existed, she was fit as a fiddle. But she was also emotionally vulnerable and could easily be coaxed by her beloved grandson.

*****

One afternoon a week into my classes, the phone rang. It was Mom, but she was not calling with the expected progress report.

"Are you sitting down, honey?" Mom asked quite calmly as I fixed an afternoon snack.

"I'm OK, Mom," I replied tentatively, hunting for the crackers.

"No, you better sit down," she said a bit more forcefully.

"OK, let me have it," I said, heading for the den, my appetite suddenly gone.

Chapter 3. The Price Tag

"The sheriff and a DEA agent came here this morning to talk to Luke."

"The DEA? The sheriff?" I cried out, falling onto the sofa.

"Yes, honey. Calm down. The agents had just come from the doctor's office. The kind man had refused to sign a complaint regarding a forged script by Luke. As a matter of fact, the doctor stood up for Luke, stating the severity of Luke's accident. He told them he was amazed Luke lived through it. He was given high doses of morphine in the hospital, only to be released without a managing physician and three days' worth of meds."

"Facts, Mom—tell me the facts," I blurted out, wishing I had grabbed the wine from the fridge.

She went on calmly. "It appears Walgreens has a forged script from when Luke was first out of the hospital."

My head was spinning. "Oh my God, Mom … how did he get to Walgreens three weeks out of the hospital?" I didn't know one could order prescription pads on the Internet.

"Yarrow probably filled it, not knowing it was a forgery," Mom said apologetically.

My heart sank. I'm sure my blood pressure was over 200/120, and my head throbbed. "Go on," I told her.

"The sheriff said the doctor spoke very highly of Luke and said that he had faith in him to regain a good life and that he was not a dope-chasing kid without a purpose. Of course, the sheriff and nice DEA man wanted to see Luke for themselves, but I told them they'd have to wait until he woke up."

"You did what?" I gasped.

"I made them tea, the green matcha type I like so much, and told them about Luke and the accident for about a half hour while he was napping. Oh, I also showed them the CaringBridge site with the posts from all his friends from church and his three-inch medical records."

"Is he in jail?" I blurted out in sheer panic. My stomach was in my throat by this point, and I was barely breathing.

My mother tried to keep me calm. "Luke finally woke up, put on his brace, and spoke with them. He even showed them his scars. They saw I was telling the truth and didn't ask him any more questions but rather extended their sympathies and commended him for struggling to get off narcotics as soon as possible. They strongly cautioned Luke of the opioid epidemic and reiterated the problems with this medication."

"Is that all?" I said with great hesitancy.

"Well, they did share heartbreaking stories of lives lost, telling Luke they spend most of their days on those kinds of calls. I think Luke got the message after they scolded him and warned him not to do it again. Luke promised he never would. We all said a prayer and shook hands. As they left, they closed the case and wished him the best."

I was lying flat on the sofa by now. "Thank you, Mom. I owe you. He could have been arrested and taken away to spend the next 15 years in prison."

"I know, honey. Have faith," she said, still in complete control.

"Mom, please, the both of you just lay low and take things easy until I get back, OK?"

"We're doing just fine. Don't you worry. I have some fun things planned for us, and I am keeping a good eye on him," my mother said confidently.

As she hung up the phone, I took off my shoe and hurled it at the ceiling, calling to God at the top of my lungs. "Stop it! Just stop it, stop it, stop it! I can't take it anymore!"

By the end of the second week, Luke had a new Mac computer, a new wardrobe, and a new cell phone. Three days later, the phone rang again.

"Hiya, Momma. Guess what Grandma bought us today?" Luke blurted out with great excitement in his voice.

"Well, hi, honey, how are you too?" I said, a tad miffed.

"Oh yeah, hi. Grandma bought us a new Jaguar! We went out this afternoon and test-drove a few cars. She fell in love with the Jaguar XJL Portfolio. It's British racing green!" He rattled on about its technology when I cut him off abruptly.

"She did what? Put your grandmother on the phone!" I demanded.

My mother claimed choosing that car was her idea and her idea only. Right. This boy was a car aficionado and knew everything about each make and model since he was six. I was not fooled. Mom promised she'd only allow him to drive it slowly in the gated neighborhood.

"No, no, Mom. No driving for Luke! He is on narcotics, and his judgment is impaired," I raged, trying to keep my temper in control. *What was she thinking?* My blood was boiling, but she hung up before

Chapter 3. The Price Tag

I could scold her. Thank heavens, Yarrow was flying back to Naples the next day.

I was a wreck but kept expecting life to get back to normal. Trying to chill that night, I remembered Patty, the ICU nurse, sitting me down to explain that an accident of this magnitude affected the one involved and the entire family. She told me that from here on out, we would mark time "before the accident" and "after the accident," creating a new normal for us all. Patty saw I was in shock and operating in survival mode and gently told me that one day I would have to deal with the trauma of almost losing my child. But I didn't have time for that right now. I had to deal with my crazy family's life-and-death challenges.

The next phone call from Mom was disheartening. Luke still had not gotten off the hard pain meds, which concerned me. His neurologist suggested injections of steroids and/or spinal blocks to help, but a new local pain doctor was still upping his Oxycontin as Luke had consistent breakthrough pain.

Luke was also working with his psychologists and counselors, who were helping him overcome the emotional trauma of the accident. He had virtually no short-term memory and had gaping holes in his long-term memories. The psychologist told us that Luke had post-traumatic stress disorder, which was unsurprising. It would take more than a few weeks to deal with it, and they weren't sure he was willing or able to deal with the issue at this early stage, stating that the subconscious will let go only when it feels safe. Luke felt far from safe.

More concerning was that Yarrow had been telling me Luke's behavior was starting to remind her of the days when he was using drugs before the accident. She didn't trust the new doctor, who seemed to be upping Luke's medications again. The more he took, the more irritable and rude he got. Luke was not the same man she fell in love with; she needed her own space to figure out her future. Yarrow hoped it would be with him *if* he would get off the drugs. She could deal with his back issues and PTSD but not drugs. I didn't blame her when she told me she needed to leave.

Now I was left alone to figure out how to care for the two broken remaining members of my family, two people I loved more than life itself, but I was running on empty as I finished the term.

*****

Summer vacation for me was a complete oxymoron. When Yarrow left, the joy was also gone from the house. Luke was trying hard not to be depressed but was lonely and scared. My mother was locked in her safe mode, acting like nothing had happened, working her business online and playing hymns. I needed a plan.

Luke could now travel and was ready to try to wean himself off the drugs. He had lost Yarrow once before because of them and was unwilling to lose her again. They were talking on the phone again, which gave him hope.

My best bet was to take Luke back to North Carolina to better manage his care and get my brother to take Mom on a trip. Thankfully, he was more than happy to help. I'd have Luke home for two weeks. Hopefully, that would be enough time to figure out the next leg of this insane journey. We packed up and headed back home to North Carolina. After unpacking, we went to see Rebecca.

The drive to Rebecca's house was excruciatingly painful for Luke as she lived on an unpaved road in the country. Her farm was a familiar place where we spent many hours licking our wounds and riding horses. It took us about 10 minutes to unload. Arm in arm, Luke and I slowly walked through the front door.

"Luke!" she cried out cautiously, reaching for a hug. "I am so glad to see you!"

He held back a painful grimace but welcomed her caring embrace.

After a few minutes of pleasantries, Rebecca got right to the point. The news was not what I wanted to hear.

"Luke, you are a very complicated case. Truth be known, my friend, I did not expect you to pull through," she stated as I took out my notepad and started taking notes.

Luke was curled up on the sofa and said softly, "That's what I hear."

She went on, paging through his medical records. "OK. I am not your doctor, but from what I can assess from your chart, your needs should be addressed in the order of severity by specialists as they are linked together. Trying to pull one out from underneath the pile could have catastrophic consequences."

She sighed. "From what you tell me, Luke, your PTSD is sometimes near the critical stage."

Chapter 3. The Price Tag

He nodded, looking at the floor. "I can remember every detail of the accident—even asking the strangers to call Mom. Then I started choking and realized it was on my blood in my mouth. That's when everything went dark." His head jerked up suddenly. "But I dream about it every night! Each roll! Each turn, crashing through the side window, seeing the car careening toward me.... Sometimes I even dream no one came to help. I always wake up screaming."

I moved closer to Luke, trying to comfort him, saying quietly, "Put it out of your mind, honey. It's all over. You made it, Luke." He nodded, trying to gain his composure.

Rebecca wiped a tear from her face. After a moment, she continued, still looking at the records. She shook her head woefully, speaking directly to me, "Susan, his dosage is too high, yet he needs some relief for his back pain. It would help if you found an addictionologist to tell you when to step him off with Suboxone. To help the healing process, he needs a physical therapist with a new pain management doctor to walk him off this insane amount of 600 mg of Oxycontin."

"Six hundred?" I gasped. Luke groaned.

She said sympathetically, "I'm sorry, Luke, it's not going to feel good, but the amount you are on now would kill most people. It is uncalled for, and, quite honestly, it is criminal they put you on that much. This drug is dangerously addictive, and it has you hooked. You are severely dependent. Do you understand what that means?"

Luke nodded sadly, his eyes on the floor. I choked back my tears.

"Susan, Luke will need an adult to keep the medication under lock and key. Luke's dependency on the pain medication requires distribution by another adult to avoid abuse. Addiction is not my field, Luke is not my patient, and I can't treat him. Do you know an addictionologist?"

"No," I replied. "I'm checking to see if I can find another doctor within driving distance who offers Suboxone treatment. His last one left the state."

Rebecca nodded her approval. "Good. He's going to need someone good."

"What about his PTSD? He's on Xanax, three bars a day."

"Who in God's name is giving him that much when he is still on high doses of narcotics?" Rebecca demanded.

"His pain management doctor," I replied. Luke held up his bottle as proof.

She just shook his head in disbelief. "Listen to me, both of you. You've got to be very careful. Xanax is very addictive, has a short half-life, and gets into the brain quickly. The effect is gone in four to six hours, causing severe withdrawal. Narcotics cause sedation. When used simultaneously with benzodiazepines, sedation can be severe, leading to respiratory depression. In the case of benzodiazepines, like Xanax, Ativan, and Valium, overdose and withdrawal can be lethal."[6]

Dear Lord, what are we dealing with? I muttered to the heavens.

"That means you could die, Luke," she said sternly, looking at us both. "Even though a doctor wrote you these scripts, they can be lethal unless you are very careful. You need to be under better medical supervision!"

"I'll keep the meds in my care until we find someone, Rebecca," I said, holding out my hand to get Luke's medications back.

Tenderly, Rebecca leaned over and told Luke, "Son, you will need rehab one day. You must get off everything and stay that way if you ever want to have a life again."

Luke started crying. "I'm scared. I'm in pain. I'm ugly and hunched over. No girls will ever look at me again. I can't think. I can't remember…"

Rebecca put down the chart and moved closer to Luke, putting her hand on his shoulder.

"One day at a time, Luke. It's only been a few months since your accident. These drugs feel like a safety net to you. I understand that. You are physically and emotionally addicted to them. But in time, they can kill you. Is that what you want?"

"No, ma'am. But I can't stop. I want to, but I just can't!" Luke exclaimed with terror in his eyes.

She turned to me. "Susan, go through the list of doctors in the North Carolina database and find one who can prescribe Suboxone and get an appointment fast. Luke, you hold on. We almost lost you once and are not about to lose you again. I believe in you!"

Luke nodded as we gathered our belongings to leave. Rebecca slowly walked us to the door, promising Luke that when he was better, we'd all go on a carriage ride together. He smiled.

We hugged, and I thanked her profusely for her help. Angels continued to show up on our path.

*****

When we left, Luke seemed relieved by Rebecca's recommendations. I was in tears with gratitude for having such an informed friend. Within days we found someone online to prescribe Suboxone. Luke would not sign the HIPPA form, so I was not allowed in the room. My fears abated when Luke walked out with a smile on his face and a new set of prescriptions. "Don't ask, don't tell" was a new policy in our house. After all, he was an adult, at least by the standards of the law.

Plans now had to be made regarding the summer. I needed to teach two full-day classes for a month, and I knew better than to leave Luke alone at home by himself. Meanwhile, my mother had returned from her trip with my brother. She also wanted Luke to come back and live with her. With a heavy heart, I put him on a plane with all his medications and specific instructions for my mother to oversee his dosages. My mother agreed to follow the doctor's instructions.

Silly me. No sooner did Luke get back to Naples did Grandma gave him the keys to the Jag so he could do her errands. She also gave him the key to the lockbox where she kept his meds, trusting his word that he would use them responsibly when she took her naps. None of us knew what addiction was, much less how it hijacks the brain, demanding its needs be met, whatever the cost.

With total freedom, Luke went out to find himself a new doctor of sorts. Armed with her credit card, stolen checks from her business account, and a nice set of wheels, Luke found a "pill mill" where he could get a steady supply of narcotics. He was still too afraid to go off them and face the physical and emotional pain he had pent up in his body.

"Pill mill" is a term used to describe an unscrupulous pain management clinic that prescribes large quantities of narcotics with little to no medical justification. These clinics are used primarily by persons abusing the drugs or for those whose physicians cut them loose. They are staffed by dishonest doctors who are only in it to make money.

Unbeknownst to me, at this time, Grandma was living in Drug Paradise USA—the capital of the pill mills. The primary drug dispensed during the 2000s was Oxycodone, and Florida was known as the "Oxycontin Express" as individuals throughout the United States traveled there to fill up. According to the House Hearing, 112th Congress report "Prescription Drug Diversion: Combatting the Scourge (2012)," Florida had more than 900 unregulated pain clinics and was home to 98 of the 100 U.S. physicians who dispensed the highest quantities of oxycodone. And here was Luke, right in the middle of it.[7]

As the weeks went on, Luke rarely called; when he did, he was evasive and rude. I suspected he was out of control, yet Mom kept assuring me all was okay. She had her grandson to fuss over and went back to her routines. I was in the last week of teaching the summer term and could not drop everything to go back down. More than that, I was not wanted. Mom told me Luke was an adult and I needed to back off and let them live their lives. She was teaching him to run her Shaklee business and was fully content with the present arrangement. The more I argued, the more she hung up.

My gut told me Luke was in trouble. Baxter was not any help either. He was sure Luke was not addicted—not his son. I became pretty persistent despite their evasions and finally got through to my mother's friends, who expressed concern for his drug usage and suggested an intervention. My mother had a better solution and took him to a prayer healing service. She called me later that evening and proudly announced that Luke was healed, so I no longer had to worry about it. Bless her heart…

Only when she got her bank statement three days later, with checks he forged for more than $2000, she called, asking me to come back down.

The severity of Luke's addiction had finally sunk in. I sobbed, remembering my son before this drug came into his life: bright, talented, funny, intelligent, and full of life. I was much more fearful of this drug claiming his life than I ever was when I stood over him in the hospital and the doctors told me he could die.

I couldn't take anymore, and I put the last few days of class on Blackboard and headed off again to Florida. With only a few weeks until the fall term, I knew I had to act fast to find the best long-term solution for them both. I dropped Katie off at Baxter's and hit the road. The 12-hour drive surely would give me some ideas.

When I saw Luke, he was thinner than ever, had dark circles under his eyes, and walked painfully with his brace and a cane. I was livid with my mother. How could she think he could be out driving, putting lives at stake, much less giving him transportation for his drug habit? She seemed oblivious. Mostly I was embarrassed and wildly angry at myself for thinking such a living situation could work out. *What was I thinking?!*

We had a major family powwow that night. I tried to get him to go to drug counseling. He would not, and I could not force him against his will since he was legally an adult. I also could not threaten to cut Luke off as Grandma would only break down to his charms again and enable him to do what he wanted. I had to use his loneliness and love of Yarrow as motivation, so I promised him I would see if the private college, 45 minutes from my house in North Carolina, would accept him for the fall semester. It had a special disabilities program which could be a perfect fit. The university where Yarrow would be going was three hours away.

That seemed to do the trick. Luke would get clean, be in college, and be close enough to Yarrow to see her on the weekends if she would take him back.

Now for the hard part. The detox. Luke broke down in tears and begged me to help him get off the medication. He confessed he was now shooting up to get the same relief pills had given him before. I was mortified. I am sure he would have overdosed if not for his high genetic tolerance.

The next 10 days of detoxing were tough on him. No one there could prescribe Suboxone. Few doctors had even heard of it, and no rehab would take him even if he were on it as they considered it "still using." I didn't know that a self-monitored detox could kill him.[8] I mean, this drug addiction situation does not come with a manual. Luke spent long days sweating in a dark room, unable to answer calls or do much of anything really except shake and fight anxiety demons. His physical pain was also exacerbated because the drug's rebound effects took hold. I sat quietly beside him, prayed … and tried to breathe myself as I washed his sweat-drenched sheets twice daily. After almost losing him in the accident, I would not lose him to drugs. Mom called on her prayer warriors. She finally saw the truth of what was happening.

When Luke was on his feet again, we found a place where there was a Narcotics Anonymous meeting every hour on the hour 24/7 for those needing support. He was there twice a day. I drove and waited in the car to ensure he did not take any detours.

Of course, without the pain protection, his energy level dipped, but his cognitive processes were much more robust. He sounded so alert, funny, and bright again. It was as if a massive ray of his light was spilling out and over. We would go to our favorite ocean bench daily and take in the healing breezes. Maybe a promising future would ride in on one of them.

The college's admittance office returned my call, saying they would consider Luke if he came to the campus and met their ACT requirements. No matter what, he was coming home with me.

With tears in Grandma's eyes, we pulled out at dawn. My heart was also breaking, leaving her alone. She refused treatment for her cancer, claiming she was in spontaneous remission, but I knew better. Reason demanded we all should be together, but when did reason ever win with us? My mother stubbornly refused to leave her home, and deep in my heart, I understood. She had always been strong, independent, and self-sufficient. Her Shaklee business kept her busy and her Lord kept her safe. It was useless to argue with her anymore.

*****

Luke slept most of the trip, thank heavens. The next day I drove him to the college, where he took the test. They scored it on the spot. His scores were high enough, and he was accepted! I jumped for joy, and he was thrilled to get a chance to have a normal life. I'd worry about the $30,000 tuition later—student loans, most likely.

Later in the evening, however, I found more pain meds in his suitcase. My heart broke. He couldn't do both and must choose. I still believed that getting off drugs was just a matter of will. A great day crashed and burned because of a drug. *Am I throwing money away? Can he ever stay clean? Will he wind up in jail, dead, or on the street?* I had yet to know that detox was not a one-shot deal for sobriety. It was chemically impossible for Luke to stay sober alone without understanding his disease, building a support team, and developing a long-term program to heal his brain.

Chapter 3. The Price Tag

How I hated the fights. I was not arguing with my son but with drugs that had control of him. Luke knew it, too, and was fighting with all he had to get off them, but the cravings were so intense. I suggested we call his doctor for Suboxone, but Luke vehemently refused to see him again. I assumed it was because he was embarrassed that he had relapsed. Luke said he knew of a new doctor closer to home who could now write for Suboxone. I did not know how he found this man, nor did I know better than to ask when he showed me the Suboxone strips and promised to wean himself off in time.

Luke was sober and acting like himself, all things considered. He and Yarrow were talking again, planning to meet during the holidays. That was his motivation. Phew. I could finally relax.

Luke and I had a great day shopping for his dorm room two days before school started. Grandma gave me money to ensure he had everything he needed. The next day we had our weekly appointment with his new doctor to regulate his Xanax now that he was off all narcotics. Luke had always suffered from severe anxiety, even as a child. The doctor told us he was dual diagnosis and would need anxiety drugs as well as Adderall for his ADD. I argued for the Adderall but was assured the Xanax would keep the Tourette's at bay. Luke was 19. The choice was his. So be it.

The next day Baxter and I took him to college and helped him get set up in his room. Convocation was that evening. It was a special night watching Luke take the oath of academic integrity with all the robed professors shaking each student's hand. Luke instantly made new friends. For the first time, my tears were tears of joy.

I wanted Luke to settle more than anything and was willing to take on debt for him if he could have a successful experience in college. His anxiety was of concern as was his back pain. Of course, drug dependency was the top concern, but it did seem to be under control.

I knew he must be the one to want to make life work, however. Luke showed us his class schedule with great pride before we left. It looked manageable. Time would tell. This time, however, I was skipping the Pollyanna routine. It was life. There would be successes and failures—mountaintops and valleys.

It was also time for me to go back to school. I began teaching my classes with new hope. It was short-lived as my cell phone rang on my way home. A doctor introduced himself to me as Luke's physician. My name was down as an emergency contact. My heart was in my throat.

The doctor was livid. Unbeknownst to me, Luke forged yet another script on some dark web script pad. By sheer grace, the doctor did not turn Luke over to the police. The doctor sternly warned me that he would turn Luke in if one more falsified script appeared in the system. He then relayed the message that BCBS had him red-flagged. From now on, any and every prescription for Luke would be sent to an open file for instant viewing. They would immediately know if Luke was doctor shopping. They would also monitor hospital ED visits. Any red flag would be instantly reported, and all past files would be opened.

In a panicked rage, I drove to Luke's school, unloading on him instead of going home. He was sufficiently scared and willingly listened to my tirade.

"Thank you, Momma. I don't deserve you. I should have died for all the pain I have caused you," he said with his eyes on the floor.

"Don't ever say that! You are my son, and I love you more than life itself—but damn it, Luke, you could go to jail! What were you thinking? You are not a criminal at heart—I know that!" I was horrified at the thought.

"No, I'm just an addict, Mom … I'm a worthless addict," he said hopelessly.

My heart broke for him. "Son, you are far from worthless! Your brain chemistry is changed; it now depends on this horrible drug![9] You've just got to do all you can to stop!" I replied, trying to salvage his self-worth, remembering the drug campaign of the 1980s: "Just Say No."

"I am trying!" he sobbed. "I love you so. I don't mean to hurt you, Mom. I can't explain why I can't just stop. I try. Every day I promise myself this is the day I will stop everything. Then I cave in."

*****

For the first time, I started to see that blaming an addict for his disease was the same as blaming someone with diabetes for their disease. Drugs had rewired Luke's brain. One can't "just say no" to a bio-neurological response that tells you that you will die without them.[10] Yet it was so confusing trying to understand addiction was not a moral failing. Unfortunately, stigma still drove that bus from 1939. The problem was I honestly had no true understanding of this monster. Clues seemed only to be lurking in the shadows of a blazing campfire on a dark, moonless night.

"We'll figure it all out, son," I said, praying to God I could.

"Promise?" We held hands.

"Yes. I love you, Luke, more than life itself. We're a team, but you are the one who must do the heavy lifting. I can't do it for you as much as I want to."

"Please don't give up on me," he said quietly.

"Never. Never, Bug. You're all I've got." I reached out to hold him.

"Grandma too," Luke reminded me.

"Yes, and Toto too."

I left Luke's dorm room exhausted but hopeful. He dodged another bullet. Being on Suboxone, he felt he could stay the course. I told him he had no choice. He swore no more fake scripts were floating about. I had to trust him. I mean, what were my options? He had none.

As the term progressed, all was quiet, drama-wise. Luke came home most weekends. We took our weekly trips to his doctor, went to dinners, and enjoyed an occasional movie.

His grades by midterm were OK. He was not getting A's, but he wasn't failing either. Reports from his professors were that he could process information well with stunning dialogue on the subject. His memory, however, was problematic. Even with extra time on tests, he struggled to retrieve the information he had just discussed.

I thought all would be okay until his doctor switched him to Clonazepam. For some reason, that drug caused Luke to get very sleepy. I suspected he was taking too much as excuses started coming in about him losing the script or having the scripts fall into the commode. The doctors reluctantly filled them as they saw he was trying hard and still not dealing with his PTSD. We sought counseling at his school, but it was apparent that no one was equipped to deal with those issues. Again, I was clueless that PTSD was an automatic cellular trauma response that bypassed the brain's control center.[11]

Luke's dean called me in mid–November to say a few of his professors were concerned about him. He fell asleep in class and was not turning in his assignments. Although he had passed all his midterms, he was missing more and more classes. The dean was genuinely concerned for his well-being. No one had seen him in the cafeteria or on campus for days.

Panicked, I left my campus and headed straight for his dorm room. *In what state will I find him? Did I make a mistake thinking he could really handle school so soon after his accident? Would he be alive?* My mind was preparing me to find him dead in his dorm room. Numb. I was numb—that was the only way I could drive without screaming. Terrified, placing one foot in front of the other with deliberate care, I made my way to his room.

I knocked on his door for 10 minutes. No response. Frantically, I searched for a resident advisor to open the door for me after proving I was his mother. The lights were off, yet I could see him lying in bed. Pushing my way through empty junk food bags and beer cans, I saw he was barely breathing. *Thank God…*

I shook him softly, evoking a slight stir. "Son, I want you to get up and get in the car. We are going home."

Luke didn't put up a fight. I kept trying to brace him as he struggled to his feet, weaving back and forth. Thankfully the car was close by. Straight away, I drove to the nearby Emergency Department to ensure he was not overdosing. After an examination, the medical staff told me he was zoned out on benzodiazepines. It was time for inpatient rehab, or he would surely die.

Chapter 4

Tough Love

"One of the most courageous decisions you'll ever make is to finally let go of what is hurting your heart and soul."
—B. Nicole

Jim Hayes once said, "A good friend will help you move. But a best friend will help you move a dead body." Sarah was that friend. She had also been my sanity for years.

Sarah and I met in community theater doing the play *Steel Magnolias*; I played M'Lynn, she was Ouiser. After the play closed, we continued our off-stage friendship as if we had known each other forever. It was natural I would call her in a time of crisis, which was usually on a weekly basis. Sarah never had children of her own but lost a favorite nephew in a car accident some years before and had adopted Luke. He called her Auntie Mame, and she lavished him with the same love and devotion as she once did her lost boy.

It was past midnight when Luke was released from the hospital. On the way home, I called Sarah to explain the latest mishap, just needing to hear her voice to tell me all would be OK. Five minutes after I tucked him in bed, the doorbell rang, and there she stood in her bathrobe and fuzzy slippers, carrying two bottles of an awfully expensive Merlot. My God, I loved that woman.

We set up camp on the sofa, scouring the Internet to find Luke a good treatment center. Not knowing where to look, I found one that looked promising according to its pictures. By daybreak, we had a bed secured for him. The treatment center had approved our insurance, and Sarah had put down the $7000 co-pay I didn't have. I just couldn't ask my mother for another penny. I was to pay Sarah back by picking up our lunch tabs from here to eternity.

By 9 a.m., we had packed the car, and Luke and I headed for RDU to get him on the plane to Miami, where the treatment center staff would meet him at the gate.

Luke was sad to leave that morning but happy to be given a chance to regain sobriety. Auntie Mame kissed him goodbye and slipped him a $100 bill as he got to the car.

"You're not helping, toots," I scowled at her as I held my hand out to Luke, demanding it back.

Luke returned it reluctantly. Sarah then promised to double the amount when he got out. I just shook my head.

"Save it for the spring term," Luke shouted to her as he climbed in the car. "Mom said I can start school all over in January without penalty!"

She raised an eyebrow.

"Luke has a medical release, so this term's grades would not be on his official transcript," I remarked, trying to keep her in her loop.

"Did they forgive his tuition too?" Sarah questioned with a grin.

"I wish," I replied, realizing I had just spent $15,000 with nothing to show for it except my stupidity at thinking he was ready to tackle college.

Sarah was waiting for me at our usual meeting place for a late lunch. Walking in, I saw a group of women from town at a table in the corner. I caught the eye of one mother, but she quickly turned away, subtly clearing her throat to alert her cronies to my presence. Heads leaned in. Eyes darted and whispers bounced through sips of iced tea. There they sat, smug, whispering in pious harmonies. I knew the cocoon of stigma they wove was really a steel cage filled with parrots. My ego was too bruised to care anymore. Besides, I knew what their kids were doing unbeknownst to them. In a strange way, I felt a sense of pity. Wisdom passed by their gate uninvited as karma sat down outside to wait. They likely wouldn't hear her rise until it was too late.

"Let it go, Susan," Sarah chided gently as she watched the exchange.

I simply nodded in agreement, trying to salvage lunch. Yet, I didn't relax until the treatment center nurse called early evening, telling me Luke was safely in their care. Then I called my mother with the news and crashed.

*****

Family members were strongly encouraged to participate in Luke's 28-day residential program. Since I could not be there in person, our interactions had to be by a weekly phone meeting. The treatment team had called Luke's father, but he refused to participate. Baxter was adamant Luke was not addicted and would get better on his own when his body healed. A part of me so wanted to believe he was right. Again, my gut told me I needed counseling as much as Luke did, so I signed up for their program.

At this point, everything I learned about drugs and addiction came from my experience working at the treatment center in the 1980s. A lot had changed since my lectures to "just say no." Thankfully, the medical community now accepted that addiction was a disease that could not be cured with willpower or nagging.

Until now, my emphasis had been on the number of drugs Luke was using and his deviant behavior. I had not yet realized how I was being affected by or even enabling his drug use. It was so different sitting on the other side of the table where I once had been terribly judgmental.

My first call with the counselor was simple. I read the information the treatment center sent about addiction and codependency. *Believe it. Ingest it. Connect the dots.* I did, and the harsh reality hit me like a ton of bricks. For the first time, I saw the actual severity of what we were dealing with—a life-threatening disease that would be with Luke for the remainder of his life. Something at that moment told me I had come face to face with my greatest nemesis; the devil drugs might just win and take Luke from me. *No. Not my boy. Not my baby...*

Soon I was back on my own. Sarah and her semi-estranged husband, Frank, were off on a three-week cruise to try to work out the problems in their marriage. Sarah had not been feeling well and was hoping that fresh air and sunshine would help her get her mojo back. I did not notice her weight loss as she was constantly dieting.

It was good that Sarah was leaving as finals needed to be graded, the children's Christmas service had to be rehearsed, and I had more lessons to learn from the treatment center about being an enabler.

In week two, we delved into co-dependency. I looked it up in *Webster's Dictionary* to see if the term truly applied to me. "A psychological condition or a relationship in which a person with low self-esteem and a strong desire for approval has an unhealthy attachment to another who is often controlling or manipulative." Ouch! I fought the fact that I was the poster child and fit the dictionary profile to a tee. It hit hard that I was enabling Luke to continue to use drugs even though I swore I wasn't. Busted!

Watching someone you love struggle with a disease like chemical dependency is hard. A mother's natural tendency is to try to fix her child's problems. At least it was mine. Luke was no longer a child, however. My angst at almost losing him in the accident made me hypervigilant and super controlling, trying to save him from drugs. This behavior had to stop for both of our sakes.

Week three's lesson plan was by far the most essential tool for moving forward. It was titled "Understanding the 'Three C's' of Personal Boundaries."[1]

I was embarrassed to find out that I had no personal boundaries regarding my son because of the guilt from the accident and my tendency to try to fix him. I also came to see I tried to fix anyone I came in contact with who appeared to need fixing—a control issue, to be sure. The feeling of control gave me a false sense of safety. Nonetheless, it was time I put boundaries in place for both of us.

Lesson: When in crisis mode, ask yourself the Three C's.

First C: Did I cause it? If the answer is no, let it go.

One of the most important things I had to learn about Luke's addiction is that I did not cause his addictive behaviors. That didn't mean he was not going to blame me. He tried many times, and I bought it hook, line, and sinker. I needed to understand what was and what wasn't under my control. My first assignment was to set healthy boundaries and help him in his journey to recovery but not buy into his bullshit when my instincts told me differently.

Second C: Can I cure it? If the answer is no, let it go.

Addiction is a chronic disease, like diabetes or hypertension, and requires guidance from a medical professional, not a Google search or Grandma's bedside reading material.[2] Addressing addiction requires both physical and mental lifestyle changes. Treatment options may include medical management of withdrawal symptoms, MOUD (medications for opioid use disorder), cognitive behavioral therapy, a strong support system like AA or NA, and residential rehabilitation.

Chapter 4. Tough Love

Third C: Can I control it? If the answer is no, let it go.

This C is a biggie. My Lord, I wish I truly understood this concept, but as a control queen, it took me a long time to relinquish my crown. Again, I always wanted to take control of Luke's addiction and anything else in his life. He always called me a helicopter mom. After all, I was a professor and was expected to have all the answers. Nothing like trying to teach astrophysics with a copy of *Dick and Jane Go to the Planetarium*.

Until this point, the onus for sobriety was put heavily on the addict—if they didn't clean up their act and stop using, they were weak and immoral. I am ashamed to say I tried to control Luke through that kind of guilt. Very few people understand that addiction, now called substance use disorder (SUD), is a bio-neurological disease affecting the brain's chemistry. Brain chemistry dictates behavior. Put jet fuel in a regular car engine, and you'll have a problem.

*****

Thank heavens, Christmas was around the corner, and we would all be together again. In years past, waiting for Grandma and Grandpa Joe to fly in for Christmas was almost as exciting as waiting for Santa on Christmas Eve. Luke and I would anxiously wait at the bottom of the escalator at RDU for them to make their grand entrance. Mom would lead the way in her pink silk fur-trimmed hoodie, carrying only her purse. Joe was behind her as the pack mule loaded with carry-ons and packages, shouting, "Ho-ho-ho!"

This year I stood alone by the elevator, waiting for the gate attendant to roll my mother in a wheelchair to baggage claim. She looked weary and frail. So did that gate attendant, loaded with her bags and paraphernalia. So much for limits for an old lady's carry-on bags. We managed to load her in the car and took off for home.

Luke would be coming home in a week, so Mom and I had plenty of time to get caught up. She always took over my bedroom when she came to stay as I couldn't put her on the sofa. Luke's room was ready for him as always, but I nailed his windows shut from the outside this time, just in case, totally forgetting the lesson of not trying to control his behavior.

While readying for bed one night, I walked in on Mom when she was taking off her shirt. She didn't try to cover her right breast. It was the size and texture of a flattened-out grapefruit.

"Mother! I thought you said you were getting better."

She was quiet for a minute, then said, "We're not going to tell Luke, Susan. I'm not in any pain, and I refuse chemo. At my age, it's slow growing, and I'm likely to die of other causes before this takes me down."

I started to cry as another painful reality hit me in the gut.

Mom hugged me and said, "Listen, Susi, I've had a good life. Better than most. There are only two things I want right now. First is for Luke to get healthy and then for you to find a good man."

"Mom, please, let me find you a good doctor. Perhaps we can turn this around," I pleaded.

"Respect my wishes, or I will leave," she said quietly. I knew her well enough to know when her mind was made up.

Luke's counselor called three days before he came home, telling me they thought Luke would be better served staying in their outpatient center for another 60 days.

"We don't think he's ready to come home, Susan."

"It's Christmas! You said this was a 28-day program," I protested.

"I know it's Christmas," she quickly replied, "but he really needs to be here and transition to the sober apartments next door for at least 60 more days. Maybe even live here permanently to be close to the group."

Without hesitancy or rational thought, my codependency kicked in gear.

"No, I'm flying him home as planned. Twenty-eight days are enough. He needs to get on with his life," I flatly responded.

"He wants to come home too, and we can't stop him. Just know we are here for you," sighed the counselor before she hung up.

I honestly thought I was doing the right thing. After all, Luke swore he was a changed man and had learned a lot—especially about the 12 Step program. He promised he'd never do another drug as long as he lived. Mom swore Luke was healed, and we would never have any more problems. Baxter swore he never had a drug problem. I drifted back into fantasy land, forgetting all the months of training and warnings. Denial can be such a sticky wicket. I just wanted my boy home.

Acting against medical advice, Luke came home in time for

Christmas. I invited Baxter to come to the airport to pick Luke up and go Christmas shopping with us at South Point Mall. Since Luke's accident, we both decided to put Luke's happiness before our differences. It helped as Luke's anger at his father's choice of an airplane over him started to ease a bit after he saw how attentive his father was to him after the accident. It was a complicated relationship. Love and hate are often close walking companions.

Our tradition over the years was to do our Christmas shopping together and finish the night by eating at P.F. Chang's. With Grandma being so fragile, we plopped her on a bench in front of Nordstrom, where she served as our package drop-off point. Luke rarely left her side except to run into a few stores. How she loved her boy. How I loved them both.

Much to my delight Christmas Eve was magical. My Christmas present to my mother each year was singing "O Holy Night" at the late candlelight service. Through the darkness, I saw Luke and Mom huddled together in their usual spot—minus Grandpa Joe. That night, joy, grief, gratitude, fear, and hope were all laid at the Christ Child's manger. Gone was the anticipation of shiny trinkets under the tree. All that was precious to me was there in front of me. Holy moments and grace.

It was a quiet drive home as we were all lost in our thoughts. Mom retired early, and I took Katie out for a walk under the stars before bed. I needed time to process my swirling emotions and change gears. Santa was coming in the morning, you know.

*****

The holidays flew by, and with tearful goodbyes, we put Grandma on the airplane on January 2. She wanted to go home to her life, and we needed to see what the new year would bring. I promised to visit her with Luke during spring break. As frail as she was, her spirit was still strong, and she was very much in control of her life.

At first, the days home went smoothly, with Luke attending daily meetings. I hesitated to return him to college, but he wanted to try again. We agreed he'd have a dorm room, but he was to spend four nights a week with me so he could go to local meetings. It all looked so good on paper.

Luke appeared changed and yet unsettled. He never spoke much about his near-death experience in the hospital. Still, he occasionally posted referencing it—as if to remind himself it was not a dream. Recovery would be challenging, but it would be possible. First, he had lessons to learn. I was trying to walk a very fine line respecting his manhood yet acknowledging that his brain chemistry was significantly compromised by the onslaught of drugs, plus his pull to continue using to feel safe.

Soon, however, I began to see cracks in his veneer and feared my decision that 28 days had not been enough considering the severity of his addiction. Sometimes one round of chemo works with those who have cancer. Sometimes a few rounds are required. I was starting to see the same holds true for SUD.

Luke's legs gave out. On January 19, 2011, at 1 p.m., Baxter called me, saying Luke was in jail. He was arrested for a DUI, blowing three times the legal limit. Baxter drove to my house so we could go to bail him out.

"I'm not doing drugs, Mom, I promise! They also gave me a drug test, which came back clean," Luke cried out as we walked into the police station.

"You can't drink, Luke!" I screamed. "It's poison to your brain. I swear, you have one beer, and you break out in handcuffs! When will you learn?"

Baxter, however, did not get the message. "Son, if you're going to drink, never get behind the wheel. Get a cab as I do."

"What?" I almost hit him.

Every part of me wanted to send Luke to his dad's and just let them go down the toilet together.

"You, Baxter, you will pay his bail and get an attorney. I'm done," I snarled, walking out to the parking lot to cry.

As January whimpered out, February blew in a blizzard of chaos.

Mid-month, Luke decided to go to New York City to visit Yarrow for her friend's birthday party. Since he didn't have a car, he hitchhiked, unbeknownst to his father or to me. I didn't even know he was gone until Yarrow called me in tears at midnight, telling me Luke showed up drunk—embarrassingly drunk—and ruined the party by throwing up on everyone. She kicked him out and apologized profusely but said she could never be with a man who acted like that. They were done!

Chapter 4. Tough Love

"Where is he now?" I asked, trying to wake up and take in the reality of this living nightmare.

"Out on the street!" she shouted before slamming down the phone.

Panic set in. Instantly I called his phone. It went straight to voicemail. *How could he pay for this trip?* Reality struck again as I fumbled through my purse to find my credit card missing. My heart sank as I knew little credit was on the card after Christmas. I logged on to my account in a daze to check for charges. A liquor store charge was all that was posted.

My heart was pounding. My son is in New York City on the street alone, drunk, and without money or any means of communication or transportation. *What could possibly go wrong?* Desperately I called all the local hospitals. No one would give me any information. The police would not consider him missing for fewer than 48 hours. I sank into my office chair, clutching my Golden Retriever, praying for his safety. And a miracle.

At 3 a.m., Luke called in tears. He was trying to find a homeless shelter, but he was too zoned out to make much sense other than a warning his phone was almost dead. Suddenly he cut out. When I tried to call back, it again went straight to voicemail. My head was burning with fear. My only comfort was knowing he was alive!

Dear God, protect him, please! was my constant mantra.

As dawn came, I canceled my classes, praying he'd find a way to charge his phone and call back. He did.

"Can I come home, Momma? I screwed up big time," he whimpered.

Thank you, God, escaped from my heart.

"Yes, Luke. Go to the bus station and buy a ticket. Call your dad so he can send you some money. *Do not hitchhike!* And call me every hour, so I know you are OK. We'll talk when you get back," I sputtered with as much calm as I could muster.

My heart, however, was pounding in my chest. I wish I could not care and disassociate my emotions from the situation, but I could not.

Twelve hours later, his father picked him up from the Fayetteville bus station. Instead of bringing him home, he drove him back to college as Luke didn't want to come home to face me. Anger exploded in my gut, but I bit my tongue. My controlling nature wanted to go after them both. But I was too exhausted. Instead, I merely thanked Baxter and hung up the phone, relieved Luke was safe.

Settling back in my chair, I remembered my codependency coaching session. This event was a situation I did not cause, could not change, and could not control. *Let it go*, whispered a voice in my head. *But how?* answered my heart. Luke was my son, my only child, and he would die without help. And so would I if I didn't learn to get a grip on the reality of the situation.

With a calm that can only come from a higher power, I reached for the Serenity Prayer. It is not just for those afflicted with the disease of SUD but also for those who love them.

> *God grant me the serenity to accept the things I cannot change, the*
> *courage to change the things I can, and the wisdom to know the difference,*
> *living one day at a time; enjoying one moment at a time;*
> *taking this world as it is and not as I would have it;*
> *trusting that You will make all things right if I surrender to Your will;*
> *so that I may be reasonably happy in this life*
> *and supremely happy with You forever in the next. Amen.*
> —Reinhold Niebuhr

*****

Luke tried to attend classes for the next two weeks but failed miserably. His dean thought it would be best for him to cut back on his course load and stay with me. We arranged our schedules, trying to salvage the term. It worked for a few weeks, but the writing was on the wall.

In the meantime, my guilt took over. I knew I had made a terrible mistake not leaving Luke in the treatment center program. Tuition was paid in full, and Luke was determined to stay on campus to make a go of classes. My trying to control him was useless. *When would that message really sink in?* I enabled him by paying the tuition for my wants, not his needs. Yes, I had learned that lesson with the Three C's, but putting them into practice was entirely another matter.

At the end of the month, I walked into Luke's room at home to find a large, and I mean huge, bottle of Oxycontin 80s on his dresser. Luke's name was on the bottle, and the date was current, but something didn't feel right. Doing a fast Internet search, I found the very same doctor who wrote the script also owned a methadone clinic right next door to his family practice. The man was creating his own addicts to profit from the methadone treatment. He didn't care, and it was legal.

In a quiet rage, I called Luke into the hall, threatening to turn the doctor in while showing Luke I had his pills. He lunged to grab them, but I spun too quickly for the snatch and locked myself in my room. Much to my horror, Luke violently kicked down the door, shattering the casing. We wrestled through his curses. Eventually, he grabbed the pills from my hand and ran out of the house.

Who was this man? Where was my son? I was frozen, mind, body, and soul.

When Luke's pills ran out in March, his bike disappeared, as did his Xbox, iPad, and computer. Strangely, my spoons were disappearing too. When I found them, they were black on the backside. There was a Dremel grinding tool in his room. Still, I did not connect the dots.

One day his cousin called, informing me Luke had stopped over with some friends for a chat. After he left, her pain meds were missing from her medicine cabinet.

"I'm not calling the cops on my cousin, Susan, but you've got to know Luke is hanging with a rough crowd and is stoned out of his mind. You've got to do something, or he's going to jail or worse. I know you've been trying to protect him because of the accident, but you've got to stop making excuses for him, or he'll die. Wake the hell up!" she screamed into the phone.

Things were falling into place to break my denial, but I stubbornly held on to hope things would get better on their own. When Luke was at home, he was tired and quiet. He'd go to his room, where I assumed he was studying or playing his Xbox. One day after a walk with Katie, I came to find out he had taken the nails off the windows and was sneaking out with friends—another failed attempt of my control.

I swore I was not in denial and kept telling myself I simply did not know what to do. I was still trying logic against Luke's brain, which was totally driven by its survival, both emotionally and bio-neurologically.

Suddenly I had a sinking feeling: *If Luke's bike and toys are gone, what else could he be hocking?* I was not giving him money, and the checkbook was secure. With a sudden panic, I ran to my jewelry box. My gold necklace, a designer gold ring, and my mother's ruby and diamond heirloom ring were gone! I was devastated. My father had given it to her for their 35th wedding anniversary. Just this past Valentine's Day, she gave it to me to remember her by.

In a rage, I ran to my car and headed straight to the local pawn shop. There was my mother's ring! Thank God. The owner informed me that the other pieces were already sold. I threatened him with calling the police if he didn't sell it back to me at that moment. I had my ring back $200 later, but my heart was in pieces. I was coming close to a total mental and physical breakdown. *Where was God? Was I being punished? Would it not have been better for Luke to have died in that accident than to live a life condemned to addiction that would surely kill him anyway? Oh God, how could I even think that?!*

*****

My mother's health was stable, but I still had to keep our ever-evolving dramas from her as the news would break her heart. Time to call Sarah. Her Lexus pulled into my driveway as if she had read my mind. Perfect timing. I knew she could help me figure things out. But when she walked in the door, I knew something was wrong. There before me stood a skeleton in Prada. She had dropped another 20 pounds from her usual size 6 in one month.

"Sit down, toots—Auntie Mame has got a problem," she said, hunting around for my wine glasses.

"You OK?" I asked, knowing better and dreading her answer.

"I went to the doctor the other day and had a second colonoscopy. I kept pooping bullets and told them I was sure they missed something," she said without emotion.

"And?" I replied, helping her find the corkscrew. She poured herself an unusually large glass of wine.

"The coloscopy was clear, but the doctor ordered an ultrasound as a precaution. They found a mass on the outside of the colon, Susan. I am going in for exploratory surgery on April 15. They are pretty sure it's cancer."

"Oh honey, no…" I started to cry. "I'm here for you. You know that. What can I do for you? I'm so sorry."

"I'm not, toots. I'm done. I've been so miserable for years; death will come as a relief. You've been my only true friend in this town, and there is only so much golf one can play," she muttered as she lit up a

Chapter 4. Tough Love

cigarette and walked out to the back patio, knowing I didn't like her smoking in the house.

"Sarah! Don't say that! I need you; I love you!" I said, choking back my tears and grabbing a glass of wine, trying to keep up with her.

She reached over and patted my hand as we sat silently, staring at the budding azaleas in the backyard. Sarah put out her cigarette and finished her wine in three large gulps.

"I love you too, Susan. Don't feel sorry for me. Quite frankly, I'm relieved. I've got nothing but heartache and loneliness in my loveless golden cage. Money can't buy happiness. Trust me. I've tried," she responded flatly. "To be honest, I'm tired of fighting."

"Please try," I begged.

"I might … but I'm not hopeful. Truth be known, girl, I hope it's the worst type of cancer known to man, and I'll go quickly in Frank's arms just to spite him," she said, heading back into the kitchen to gather her belongings.

"Sarah, stay for a while. I'll make dinner," I said, hoping to talk her into a better frame of mind.

"Nope, gotta go. Listen. I didn't come over for pity. I'm just trying to tie up loose ends before next week's surgery. What I really want to talk about is Luke," she replied.

I hung my head. "He's a mess, but I think…"

Sarah put up her hand to stop my lame excuses.

"Susan, you've got your boy and a good life ahead of you both if you can get his life back on track. He's not acting this way to be a jerk. He's hooked on a substance over which he has no control. Trust me, I know," she said, pouring herself a roadie cup. "He needs long-term care. Here's a check for ten grand," Sarah said as she pulled out her checkbook.

"Sarah, I can't take any more of your money. You've been more than generous," I protested.

"I can't take it with me, kid," Sarah replied, writing the last zero. She tossed the check on the table. "Put Luke in a year-round sobriety house, and he might have a chance. Check out the ones in California. I'm from LA, and they have a much better support system for young people than they do here. It's time for tough love, my friend. If you don't wake up soon, you'll be burying us both—and you don't look good in black." She said this with a wink as she walked out my door. "Tell Luke I love him," she shouted out the car window. "I always wanted a boy like him."

That night I fell into bed sobbing and feeling totally helpless. Joe was gone. My mother had terminal cancer, and now Sarah was probably dying, leaving me without a support system. My fairy tale life was gone, leaving me shattered and defeated. I had exhausted all avenues to save my child and fell into bed sobbing, desperately pleading to God for a miracle. I saw no way out of this hell except death. *Dear God, if he is going to die, please don't let me be the one who finds him* were the last words running through my mind before drifting off. There was no longer any worry of nightmares. I was living one. The drug was winning, and I was out of options.

*****

Morning came in its usual fashion. Luke had been out late again, but at least he was home, as his car was in the driveway. *Will this be the morning?* I thought, hesitating to look in his room. Memories haunted me of a friend who went to kiss her 25-year-old goodbye one Sunday morning only to find him dead. That moment stuck in my head forever. I knew I could face the same horror any day.

Trying to build up my courage to check on him, I cleaned his bathroom. There, tucked away in a corner, was a used needle in tissue paper with what appeared to be blood on it. Instantly my denial was miraculously broken. I calmly unwrapped it and walked into his room to face the inevitable.

"Luke? You awake?" Mild stir. He was breathing, thank God. "Luke, I need you to wake up." He opened his eyes slightly.

With calmness and great clarity, I told him, "I found this used needle in the bathroom. I am not a fool. I don't know what you are shooting up, and frankly, I don't care, but I want you to know it's over. I can take getting a phone call telling me you died from an overdose. I have accepted that you will probably die, but I can't take being the one who finds you dead in our home. You have 24 hours to gather all your belongings and find a place to stay. No car. No money. No credit cards. Nothing. I will change all the locks and get a restraining order if need be. Either that or I will send you to a year-long sobriety program. The choice is yours."

With that, I shut his door and sat down at my desk, not knowing what kind of hell would erupt. It didn't matter. I was done. This was my final stand.

Ten minutes later, I heard his door open. He quietly walked into my office, wiping tears from his face, and sat in my big red chair.

"I can't stop, Mom. I don't know how to stop. I've tried everything, and I've given up. I need help so badly, but I don't know how," he sobbed.

These were real tears—absolute desperation. No one wants to continue a life of hell, yet the road out is so incredibly complicated.

"Come here, son." I reached out to hold him as he let it all out: heartache, confessions, fears, and disgust with himself.

"I can't fix this, but you can, Luke. You must commit this moment to want sobriety more than your next breath." He nodded. I went on, "You can't stay in North Carolina either. There are too many temptations here. I've been on the Internet and I see California has high success rates with its recovery programs. You move there and call California home, so your support system is always nearby," I stated authoritatively.

"Will you come to visit?" Luke asked with a sudden fear of abandonment in his eyes. I had always been his safe place. Shaking off weakness, I remembered my rescuing had to end if he was to get better.

"After a year, yes. You need to do this on your own first. I promise we'll talk all the time, but you must do this alone," I said firmly.

"OK. I can't go on like this, Mom. I don't want to die. I am powerless over my addiction, and I need help," he said, acknowledging the truth of my words. Little did we know he had just completed Step One of the AA/NA programs.

There was no instruction manual to help guide us, only the Internet. Luke and I searched for possible treatment facilities and found a well-respected program in Palm Springs. I called my insurance company, which approved the program for detox and a 35-day program with the possibility of 90 days should he need it. When I called the intake counselor, he informed me the facility couldn't accept our insurance because it was from out of state.

"But you take BCBS! My insurance company already approved it," I quickly retorted.

"Listen, lady," he casually responded, "this is how it works. In-state insurance companies send us the checks directly. Out-of-network sends you the check, and you are then supposed to send it to us—but since so many people just keep the cash, we've established a policy not to accept out-of-network anymore. I'm sorry." Click.

Luke's heart sank. Mine exploded in a rage of disbelief. My child's life was at stake. He needed immediate treatment. I was not about to back down. With the tenacity of a momma bear protecting her cub from poachers, I immediately redialed, telling Luke, "My daddy always told me that the wheel that squeaks the loudest gets the grease." The same intake counselor picked up.

"You've got to take him. He's going to die here. No one on the East Coast can help him. Trust me, we've tried," I pleaded.

"Susan, I'm sorry, we just can't break the rule. Besides, the co-pay is $10,000 upfront cash. You have that kind of money on a professor's salary?"

"As a matter of fact, I do." I didn't tell him my dying friend Sarah had recently gifted me a check for Luke's treatment. "I'll wire it to you this minute! Sir, I'm desperate. I don't want my son to die; you are his only hope!" I sobbed. "I swear, the second I get the checks from insurance, I will overnight them to you!"

The counselor softened. "One day late, he is on the street without anything. You understand that?"

"I swear on my life, sir. Without Luke alive, I might as well be dead too."

"Insurance will pay for most of the 90-day program, but then he must go into our sober living house in Palm Springs or LA. It's the only way severe addictions can get healed. His dopamine receptors need to repair, and that takes a long time. It's a rigorous program, and you can't see him except maybe for a few days at Christmas. No exceptions. You've got to sign a binding contract."

"That's what I understand, and I fully accept the terms," I replied earnestly.

The counselor got stern once again. "Insurance does not pay for sober living houses. It will cost three thousand dollars a month, upfront cash."

"Not a problem," I blurted out confidently.

Chapter 4. Tough Love

Luke looked at me as if I was crazy.

The voice on the other end paused, then finally responded, "OK, Susan. Wire the money and get him on the first flight out Sunday morning. Send us the flight itinerary. That will give you two days to pack and complete all the paperwork."

"Thank you, sir. God bless you," I whispered through my tears. Luke and I did the Snoopy happy dance together.

Luke's mood suddenly shifted, and he became somber. "I've got a small problem, Mom."

"Now what?" I asked, totally exasperated.

"I will need Suboxone to get me through the next few days, so I don't go into full withdrawal. I'm out of drugs and feel the cravings are strong."

Damn it! Why can't a regular doctor prescribe this drug?! I shouted to myself.

"It's Friday," I reminded Luke. "Can you get in to see a doctor with the waiver to prescribe it?"

"No. I don't know of any in the area," he replied.

"OK, so what do we do?" I asked in dismay.

"I can get some off the street. It'll cost about $200 for four tabs. I think I can make it on that amount."

"You can get Suboxone off the street?"

"You can get anything off the street, Mom."

"Silly me," I muttered as I spun out the dire situation in my head. There was only one option. "OK, let's get dressed and go to the bank. You make the call. Just don't tell me the details, OK?"

I had just agreed to commit a felony, yet for some unknown reason, I simply took out my checkbook.

"Auntie Mame gave you the ten grand, didn't she?" Luke asked.

"How'd you know?" I asked. Luke was aware of our financial difficulties.

"Sarah called me the other night and told me she loved me—and told me to be a good boy or she'd come back to haunt me. She looked pretty sick the other day. I kind of figured it out."

I shook my head in acknowledgment. "Come on, let's get moving here."

On the way to his room to change, Luke asked, "Hey, Mom, where will you get the $3000 a month for the sober living house?"

"I haven't a clue, kiddo, but we'll deal with that later. I've got 90 days to figure it out."

We planned to take Luke's car. I didn't want to be spotted in mine should anyone be watching. Before leaving, I donned a heavy, oversized ski coat and pulled a ski cap down low to cover my hair and hide my ears. I debated adding a fake mustache from my theater makeup kit. If I could have hidden my eyes and face, I would have. I wanted to hide but needed to show up for my son.

Luke poked his head into the bathroom to see if I was ready.

"You look silly, Mom," he said, crinkling his nose.

"Don't care," I stated flatly.

And off we went to make my first drug deal. *Dear Jesus, don't let Judgment Day come until this is over, and I will make it up to you. I promise!*

Truth be known, I was terrified. While I was getting ready, my mind played out the consequences of getting caught. I knew full well my tenured position at the university would be in jeopardy. Some church friends might understand, but I doubt they would have let me continue as the children's worship arts director. I chuckled at the irony of once being petrified of getting caught smoking a cigarette in front of my father when I was in my 20s.

Yet here I was, an accomplished woman with high standing in the community, risking everything for a drug that should be available to anyone suffering from SUD. My shame was overridden by disgust at the absurdity of it all.

"OK, son, where are we headed?" I asked, cautiously pulling out of our driveway.

"Carthage. The McDonald's parking lot close to Nana's old house," he instructed me.

"Carthage? Really?" I asked in disbelief. Carthage was a small town 15 minutes down the road. It was also the county seat, and the courthouse was two blocks from the rendezvous location. Squad cars would be everywhere. Like we were living in a scene from *Bonnie and Clyde*, I suddenly feared we might have more challenges than initially anticipated.

"Sorry, Mom. Not my call," whispered Luke as he clutched his stomach. His detox was coming on strong as I watched the sweat pour down his face.

Chapter 4. Tough Love

"Hang on, Bug," I said as I punched the accelerator.

My mind raced with memories as we cut through the back roads. Life had dealt us so many blows in the past few years. My precious Bug had his world blown up so many times by circumstances far beyond his control. I just wanted him well. Was that too much to ask?

I pulled out of the Carthage ATM, trying to maintain the speed limit. My heavy ski gear costume would be hard to explain if I got pulled over—it was spring and a balmy 84 degrees that afternoon in North Carolina.

"Over there," Luke instructed, gesturing for me to park across the street from the meeting location. "Hightail it out of there if I get caught, Momma."

No way, I thought to myself. But what would I do? Stagger out of the car looking like a bag lady, politely explaining to the officer the absurd restrictions on this life-saving drug? We would be sharing a jail cell, I was sure.

"Be careful," I cautioned Luke as he exited the car. My heart beat out of my chest as I watched him approach a group of guys drinking milkshakes. I would have missed it if I had not been looking for the subtle exchange. A high five. A hug. A fallen napkin picked up by a thoughtful friend. After a goodbye handshake, Luke returned to the car with a slight smile on his face.

"They only had three," he told me as he shut the car door and popped a pill in his mouth.

"Will that be enough?" I asked, not knowing anything about the dosage he would need to get him through to Sunday.

"Let's hope so," Luke replied.

But it wasn't enough. By Saturday afternoon Luke was breaking into a sweat. He had broken the last two tablets in half to make them last longer.

"I don't know if I can hold on, Momma," Luke admitted, the signs of detox kicking in again.

"Let's just go get some more," I suggested, pleading in the silence of my own thoughts: *Please, God, let us get through the next day and get Luke safely into the treatment center to detox.*

"There is no more in town," he said, "I've been checking all my sources. What are we going to do?"

I called a nurse friend to ask for advice. She worked in the ER. Certainly some physicians there had the X-waiver to prescribe Suboxone and she could pull a few strings.

My friend flat-out said no. The only information she shared was that only certain pharmacies carried Suboxone because it was not a common drug. She ended the call saying, "Sorry."

Still driven to get Luke on that plane, I scoured my brain for a loophole and took Luke to the local family-owned pharmacy. We pulled up to the drive-thru window and asked to talk to a pharmacist. Maybe she would know of someone. In my usual modus operandi—panic—I explained the situation. I showed her Luke's plane ticket and insurance card, the admittance papers to the rehab center, plus any other items I could think of, explaining he only had half a tab of Suboxone left. That would never get him to LA without him going into full detox, which meant he might not be allowed to board the plane. I asked, "Could you please help me find anyone who could write us a script for just two more tabs?"

The pharmacist looked down momentarily, then replied, "Can you come into the store by yourself? I need to explain something to you. I'll meet you in the back."

I nodded and parked the car, praying for yet another miracle.

The look on her face was grim. She approached the corner to meet me and said, "Mrs. Paschal, I truly understand your situation. It's a crime that this drug has such harsh restrictions when it's one of the only ones that can save people who are addicted to narcotics. But you must understand that only a licensed physician with an X-waiver can write a script by law, and no one is around to do that. Even if there is a qualified doctor here, it is Saturday, and the offices are closed. Hospital ERs don't have the drug either."

"I know. My nurse friend told me," I said, trying to keep my tears at bay.

She went on. "You have to understand, too, that if a pharmacist gave you any without a script, they could be prosecuted and lose their license for life. It is against the law."

I nodded sadly with acceptance.

"You understand what I am saying?" she said in a deliberate tone.

I nodded in defeat. "Yes, ma'am, thank you."

"Best wishes to you and your son. I'll be praying for you." She extended her hand, wishing me the best. I reached out my hand in appreciation and felt her slip something into my palm. Her eyes fixed on mine. She turned quickly and left. I walked quietly to the car with tears in my eyes where Luke waited.

"No go, huh?" He shivered.

I opened my hand and handed him two Suboxone. "Don't ask, don't tell."

"Thank you, Momma Bear."

Angels live among us. So, too, does addiction.

I wish that the compassionate act of one kind soul was enough to overcome Luke's battle with SUD. I didn't want to believe it then, but on some level, I knew a new battle was just beginning.

Chapter 5

The Circle of Life

"Every new beginning comes from some other beginning's end."—Seneca

Sleep escaped me that Saturday night. A miracle had been given to me, but it also meant I would be saying goodbye to my son, perhaps never to see him again. The helicopter mom was crashing as she no longer had a say in matters—nor even a remote semblance of control. Intellectually I knew it was for the best. My constant denial and attempts to negotiate with this terrorist called addiction were useless. I had done more harm than good. It was time for sanity.

It was difficult to look beyond my pain to do what I could to save my son's life. I wanted him home. I wanted back the time I had lost during his traumatic teen years. I wanted him healthy with a great future like all my friends' children, yet I knew he had a disease that would plague him for the rest of his life. My heart was crushed. I was numb. Grief. Fear. Anxiety. Terror. Each emotion was taking turns punching me in the gut. *I give up, God! I can't handle this anymore. I surrender. Please take the wheel—and be merciful, to him and me...*

Luke seemed calm and had a true sense of peace about him. For the first time in ages, he had hope. That night he cleaned his room and went to bed early. When Luke was ready to go in the morning, he thoughtfully closed the door behind him with one suitcase in hand. That was all he was allowed to bring—just a few clothes and toiletries. He had one Suboxone left to get him safely out to California.

He kissed Katie goodbye and thanked her for being such a good friend. She was his Christmas present when he was 10, and he had raised her as his buddy. As life goes, she grew old as he grew up. He knew he might never see her again and thanked her for all her devotion. It was

Chapter 5. The Circle of Life

a painful goodbye. Dogs know. Katie buried her head in his knees and would not move for the longest time as he stroked her back, saying, "Thank you—I luff you."

We called Grandma on the way to the airport. He wanted to be the one to tell her. She cried with joy and prayed with him.

We had one last long hug at the airport's TSA gate. We held on for dear life while trying to act normal in front of the other passengers. I tucked a handwritten note in his backpack, telling him to read it on the plane. My mother started that tradition years earlier when I left home for school. She knew I'd need something tangible to reach for when fear or loneliness crept in. Seeing the letter, Luke hugged me with loving gratitude. Of course, it was not our first letter or our last. Years later, Luke told me he collected them all in a shoe box and would pull them out on dark days.

Most mothers and sons have natural beginnings, growth, and separations. Birth to adulthood—the natural order of things. Roots to wings. Most mothers and sons, however, do not have death as a constant ghoul stalking them. Our relationship was anchored at a deeper level. It was grounded in survival. "Crisis bonding syndrome" is the term used by psychologists. We were bonded in the fight for life. His life. He needed to know I was with him every step of the way, cheering him on in his journey to sobriety. Never judging him. Never abandoning him. At the same time, I was challenging myself to learn more about the disease of SUD and how not to be an enabling parent.

Watching Luke walk out of sight gutted me. Take me on, addiction. I will be your greatest adversary. You threaten him, and you threaten me, too. You have him in your grips, but you do not have me, and I will fight for his life until my last breath. As God is my witness, you'll have to take us both to claim him.

I was now a changed woman. Life's circumstances had turned me into a warrior. No more feeling sorry for myself. No more condemning myself or others who also walked this treacherous road. I had faced my greatest fear—losing my only child. Not many things scared me anymore. My pride had been trampled in the dust, my arrogance turned into compassion, and my ignorance slowly became wisdom. I was now on a mission. Bring it on.

*****

Luke made it to California safely and detoxed in the Palm Springs medical clinic. Daily reports informed me of his body's reaction to clearing itself of the drugs. He was having a tough time with it as he had been using a combination of substances that could have killed him without medical supervision in a detox situation. His cravings were intense. This center, like most, did not believe in using Suboxone long-term. They ignored the emerging science that some people may need to be on it for years before tapering off.[1]

The day after term ended, I packed the car with a summer full of belongings and one loving, lumbering Golden Retriever. Off to Naples again. The 12-hour drive would now take 15 hours as potty stops with snacks with ball chases had to be added to the schedule. By 3 a.m. I was on the road. I liked leaving early. By the time the sun rose, I'd be well on my way. A mind game, to be sure, but one that worked.

Punching in the garage code that let me in the house was a safe way to sneak in and surprise Mom. She was in a deep sleep in her recliner. As I stood and watched her for a few minutes, I instinctively knew I should not work that summer but put all my time and attention into her care. So much for tenure and promotion. When Mom woke up, I saw my instincts were right. She had lost a lot of ground and could not do much alone.

The days slowly lumbered on. I worked on next semester's class lectures in the mornings, did errands for Mom in the early afternoon, and ended my day by taking a three-mile walk on the beach to process everything. In the evening, I'd make us a healthy dinner, then we'd read and tell stories of happier days. Mom had gotten reasonably competent at letting Katie go outside to potty and filling her water bowl. It was a win-win for everyone. I seriously thought of leaving Katie with Mom as they were getting very attached to each other, but I realized that one squirrel could end it all for them both.

It took a few days to convince Mom that she really should see a breast cancer specialist. Her tumor was turning odd colors. And I could see she was in pain. The woman had no trust whatsoever in conventional medicine, but perhaps it would not hurt to see what someone had to say this time. She eventually did not protest my making an appointment.

I escorted my mother into the medical clinic with my scribing pad

Chapter 5. The Circle of Life

but soon realized I didn't need to use it. Our physician was a good man with a kind heart. After a thorough check-up, he told her she had stage IV metastatic breast cancer—a fact she suspected but never wanted to admit. Of course, she debated the findings and presented her reasons. The doctor was a saint and listened patiently before gently guiding her back to the obvious tumors and lumps in her lymph nodes.

After moderately accepting his findings, she finally said in a resigned tone, "Well, I suppose I should consider getting it removed now." There was a long pause.

"I'm afraid it's a little too late. I'd have to remove half your chest," the doctor said as he shot me a glance insinuating *"Why did she wait so long?"* I could only shrug. To say anything more would upset her. I think he understood. He suggested we set up hospice care. We thanked him and left.

With a script for pain meds she was not about to take, we headed for the car and sat silently for the longest time. She knew I was shaken at hearing she would die soon and took my hand. "So be it. God is in control. Let's contact hospice."

I nodded and started to cry. She held me as only a mother could hold her shaken child.

"I've had a great life, Susi. Better than most—two wonderful husbands, children I love, nine beautiful grandchildren, my two schools, great friends, and my Shaklee family. It's time, and I am at peace. God has been more than gracious to me," she said with acceptance.

"OK," I said, drying my tears. "What next?"

"I need you to help me put my house in order. Can we go to the beach first? To our bench? I just want to take in the sunset."

"Of course." I needed to process everything too. There is nothing like having your suspicions confirmed. My world. My people. My mom … all leaving me.

*****

The days that followed were calm and filled with grace. Every day Mom would ask about Luke, and I would feed her info that I heard from the staff. After the first month, Luke and I could talk weekly, although Mom took up the more significant part of his allotted 10 minutes. That was OK. I had not told him her prognosis yet, but I think he knew. I

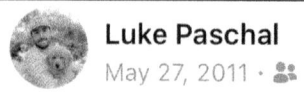

Luke Paschal
May 27, 2011

It is better to conquer yourself than to win a thousand battles. Then the victory is yours. It cannot be taken from you, not by angels or by demons, heaven or hell

Luke's post from rehab.

just enjoyed hearing him sound so strong and healthy again. His confidence was coming back, and he was gaining discipline and bonding with good role models who were guiding him through the 12 Step program of AA.

Soon he was given his phone back to make personal calls to approved people and to post messages. He called Grandma one day to tell her he had decided to turn his will and life over to the care of God as he understood Him and that he had made a searching and fearless moral inventory of himself. These are Steps Three and Four of the AA 12 Step program. We were greatly encouraged as we could see he was standing firm on his own and becoming the man he was born to be.

When we hung up, Mom enquired, "So, how are you going to pay for the sobriety house? I hear he is supposed to go at the end of June. That's only a few weeks away."

Deep breath. "You know, I was going to ask you if I could take a second mortgage out on my home—it's in the trust, you know, so I can't do it myself."

"And when were you going to ask me?" she asked.

"Now seems like a good time," I sheepishly replied.

My mother opened her handwritten ledger that held all her financial accounts. Excel was not a part of her vocabulary. She also pulled out her will and trust.

"How much can you afford to pay out of pocket?" she asked, going into her business mode.

"About $500 a month if I don't rob a bank." I half grinned.

She took some time before she spoke, paging through her ledger.

"Susi, for the past 20 years, Grandpa and I have been paying full tuition for all my other grandchildren except for Jenni. She put herself

Chapter 5. The Circle of Life

through school without my help. I'm talking thousands of dollars a month. Joe's investments are almost gone. It all adds up."

I was expecting a rejection, and that would be OK. I'd find a way somehow. My mother had given me more than my fair share over the years. I could try for a bank loan through my credit union.

She went on. "You know Luke means the world to me, and I want to be able to help him again by paying $2500 a month. One day my business and some of my personal funds from the schools and my business will be yours, and then it will go to Luke. If I die before he leaves the sobriety house, the money will be used to help him. Agreed?"

"Agreed. Wow. Thank you, Mom." I was truly amazed at her generous offer.

We went to her attorney the next day. Mom talked, and I merely listened as she dictated the changes to her will. Since Joe had died, Mom added me to the trust and named me her trustee. The final papers would be drawn up, but with her signature, it was complete as of that moment.

The end of June came quickly. Luke's insurance benefits ran out, and he'd have to move into a 12-month sobriety house. The program director called, telling us two choices Luke had to continue his recovery.

"Hi, Susan and Helene. I wanted to explain Luke's choice, so you understand the situation. Luke had two choices. The first was the house here in Palm Springs. It is an open-concept sobriety house. People may come and go at will if they test clean. They attend one organized AA meeting daily and get a job or go to school. They have house chores and rules and must obey a curfew to stay in the house."

"What was the second?" I asked, thinking the first house might give him too much freedom.

"The second house is in LA. It is closed and regimented. Participants can only go out with group leaders for the first three months and earn points for rewards and special trips. Two meetings are required daily—one in the house and the other at the local AA community meeting place. If they are on target after three months, they can get a job or attend community college. They just need to take a drug test every day when they get home. The house relies heavily on behavior modification and the 12 Step program of AA/NA. Everyone has their own individual sponsor. Together they continue to work one of the 12 steps each month for a full year until the entire Big Book is completed."

"We choose the second," Mom piped in without even looking at me.

"It's not up to you." The director reiterated, "It's up to Luke." He had already made his choice so he could be responsible for his own actions.

"What did he choose?" I asked, fearing he again chose the easy out.

"The first one. We let Luke out for 24 hours, and he came back loaded."

"Oh, no!" I sank back in my chair, devastated. Mom just hung her head.

The director continued, "Quite frankly, ladies, we knew this would happen. We needed Luke to see for himself, so he would only have himself to hold responsible. Don't be hard on him. Only 7 to 10 percent of addicts can resist the cravings after such a short time. Research suggests it takes several months for dopamine recovery to occur in mild to moderate dependencies.[2] However, the damage from severe dependency can last longer, requiring a year or even longer for the brain to recover. Some drugs can permanently damage the receptors that re-absorb dopamine, preventing the brain from fully recovering.[3] Luke has had a deluge of drugs for years. Whether his usage came from the accident or was recreational, it doesn't matter if the damage is the same. He will need a full year for the dopamine receptors to heal and hopefully return to normal. But even then, he may always have a harder struggle than others. He's predisposed to relapse in so many ways. He still won't talk about the accident and has an abnormally high anxiety level and PTSD."

"Wow. OK, I understand.... I'm just so disappointed and ashamed," I muttered.

"Shame does not work here. Addiction is a disease that comes in different levels and severities—just like cancers. Mild dependency, moderate and severe are the levels we talk about now.[4] Different substances affect the brain in different ways. Luke is severe with a very high tolerance level for alcohol, benzos, and opioids," the director said, hoping his message would sink in.

Chapter 5. The Circle of Life

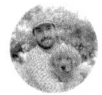
Luke Paschal
January 12, 2011 ·

before and again, I miss the voice that brought me to my knees.. my legs are so tired of standing..

Luke's post reflecting on his near-death experience.

"That I know.... Luke's father is a functional alcoholic with a very high tolerance. It is genetic," I reminded him.

Then the director dropped another bombshell. "His father wants him to come home, you know. They spoke last night."

I just gasped, "No ... please, no."

"Again, it is Luke's choice. It is his life, not yours—as hard as that is to hear, it's the only way to create accountability," the director said with authority.

Taking a deep breath while trying to regain my balance, I asked what would happen now.

The director continued, "Luke wants to recover. He chose to go to the LA house and is on his way there now. Please send a check for $3000."

"Thank you, Jesus" escaped from my mom's lips.

"It's on its way," I said as I thanked him again for his guidance and compassion.

After I hung up, Mom weighed in again. "God is good, Susan. Lessons need to be learned by individuals themselves—the director was so right. Now Luke has a chance. Never, ever, ever, ever, give up on that boy!"

"I won't, Mom. I promise," I assured her.

Mom wrote a check for the total amount, and I walked it to the mailbox. Halfway there, however, I suddenly felt guilty and very sad. I was so blessed to have a mother with money who loved us enough to pay for the care Luke needed to have a fighting chance. Our total bill with co-pays would be $36,000 that year. *What about the mothers who can't pay? Those who don't have the means—what do they do? They love their children just as much as I love mine.* After hearing the director's statistics, the reason many don't survive made sense.

After putting the check in the box, I thanked God for Mom's generosity and grieved for those left behind to fend for themselves. No parent should ever lose a child because they can't afford the treatment. It's sad that you never quite get that one until your kid's life is on the line.

*****

August was around the corner. Try as I might, Mom vehemently resisted coming to live with me. She slowly kicked into her North Dakota "chin-up" mode, although the cracks came through her stalwartness as she prepared to say goodbye. Our checklist was done after setting up hospice. care It made us both feel better that her neighbors would be there daily to check in on her.

Before I left to return to North Carolina, we talked with Luke, who was settled in his new home in Los Angeles. He loved it! There was discipline, structure, new friends, and a sponsor to whom Luke felt connected. When staff told me his bed was made daily, and all his clothes were folded neatly in the drawers, I questioned if they had the right kid. Both are part of the program. The sobriety house was in a nice neighborhood. That fact alone gave him pride and did not make him feel like an outcast, as he had experienced before in the dangerous area of the last outpatient treatment center. Luke loved the fact he was living in LA with the beach, the blondes, and real men friends. With hope settling in, I started to relax.

My mother and I said our goodbyes that night as I planned my usual 3 a.m. departure, leaving her to sleep. When my alarm went off, I found Mom waiting at the door in her bathrobe. We loaded the car and shared silent hugs, kisses, pats to the pooch, and a prayer. As I backed out of the driveway before dawn, I caught her silhouette standing in the door frame, blowing us goodbye kisses. It is a memory forever etched in my mind. Such a perfect summer. Such a gift to spend so much time walking Mom's last miles with her. By daybreak, I was headed toward Jacksonville. By 5 p.m. Katie and I were home. Unfortunately, my Sarah would not be there to greet me. She had passed away in Frank's arms three weeks earlier.

*****

Chapter 5. The Circle of Life

A few weeks after I returned home, my girlfriends were getting on my case to go out and find a man.

"Susan, you've got to get on Match.com," Caryl announced.

"No, thank you! The last time I tried that site, I had a nutcase sending me sonnets filled with political insanities and another who was not sure he'd be comfortable with a woman with advanced degrees. He liked young, buxom blondes … if you know what I mean, 'wink wink,'" I replied despondently.

"At least give eHarmony a shot," Reggie piped up. "I've known quite a few people who have found good men on that site. It screens people thoroughly. I mean, there is at least a 10-page compatibility assessment to take before it sends any names."

"Humph…. I grunted with an appropriate eye roll.

"I mean it, Susan, it's worth a try. Luke's safe. Your mom is stable. It would be better than your last date and current prospect," Reggie insisted.

Maybe they were right. My last date was with an egomaniac. The only other man pursuing me was 90. What did I have to lose? I knew eHarmony had a good reputation and would not let men have my contact information until, or if, I wanted that to happen.

"OK, ladies, I'll fill out the form tonight," I said, knowing I might get cold feet before my car left the parking lot.

Gaining resolve at home, I opened the webpage. A free week trial gave me the impetus to fill out the questionnaire. That sucker was long! It took me three days to go through all the pages as I kept chickening out. Finally, I hit "send" and said a prayer.

Next on my agenda was a fun mini-vacation without being a caregiver. My niece Jenni was flying in so we could go to the beach for a long weekend. We both needed to laugh and take a few days together. I had not seen her since Luke's accident and desperately needed my niece's loving support.

Before Jenni and I left, a picture of a man with two dogs came through the eHarmony site. *I have a soft spot in my heart for puppy dogs* was the caption under his picture. Hmmm. He was handsome, educated, a retired Major from the military, now in government service. Anyone who has a soft spot in their heart for puppy dogs might be worth a try. I gave him a "wave" on the site minutes before Jenni and I headed for the beach.

While on vacation Jim and I would wave back and forth at each other on the eHarmony site, casually letting at least one day go between relays. Neither one of us wanted to look desperate. Tentatively I then only answered the site questions—nothing very personal. Jenni was my cheerleader, and the time lag allowed me to find some courage to meet up with him in person when I got back home.

*****

Meanwhile, Luke was continuing his recovery. He called one night, telling me about his work on the next three steps of AA.

Step Five: He admitted to God, himself, and another human, which was me, the exact nature of his wrongs. Even though I survived the brunt of his misdeeds, it was healing for us both. Steps Six and Seven brought me to tears. Happy tears. He was entirely ready to have God remove all these character defects and humbly asked Him to remove his shortcomings.

That night was our first adult-to-adult conversation. Luke didn't make excuses or accusations. We merely spoke of the disease, his path to recovery, and our love for and belief in each other. After hanging up, I felt it was time to invest in my life again and start dating.

The next day Jim asked if we could perhaps have a real conversation instead of just messaging on the dating site's email. He gave me his phone number and asked me to call if I wanted to. It was totally up to me, and it was OK if we kept up the chats. I decided to take the chance with him and called during the hours he said he would be available.

Our first call went on for more than an hour. We both had roots in Michigan and knew the same haunts. We were the same age and shared the same timely memories. We both loved football and puppy dogs. We loved rhubarb pie instead of birthday cake. That was the clincher. Time to meet.

What have I done? Panic set in. My life now was calm, but I carried the dregs of war with me. Here I was with a son in rehab and a dying mother. How could I possibly think I might be able to make someone a good girlfriend? Naturally, I called Mom.

"Just be yourself, Susan. Tell him about your life—with as little drama as you can muster," Mom laughed. "If he is the right man, he

Chapter 5. The Circle of Life

will be strong enough to understand the situation and walk the journey with you. If not, you will know." She was always so wise.

Jim and I met at the Jefferson Inn, and after two hours of chatting, we agreed to go to dinner. However, as soon as we sat at the table, I started with my monologue.

"Listen, Jim, there's something I need to tell you. My life is rather complicated…"

Without taking a breath, I told him about Baxter, the bankruptcy, the terrible divorce, Luke's accident, the subsequent addiction, and the ensuing recovery progress. Lastly, I detailed my mother's condition while drawing an invisible map of events on the table.

"There you have it." I sat back, winded, and waited, fully expecting him to get up and leave.

Jim paused and then smiled. Calmly he hailed the nearest waiter and ordered a bottle of wine. "At our age, my dear, life has its complications. I look forward to getting to know you better," he said after taking a deep breath.

At the end of the long evening, we hugged goodbye, Jim promising to call the next day. He did.

The next morning's 8 o'clock check-in call with my mother was short and sweet: "Mom! He liked me!"

"I can't wait to meet him, my dear. He sounds wonderful." she responded with a hint of relief before moving on to her daily news.

Jim and I quickly took down our profiles from eHarmony and started dating exclusively. The following weeks were filled with meeting friends, walking the dogs by the river, road trips, long Saturdays of love and laughter. After 10 years of being alone, I felt the tide had finally turned in my favor. Luke was very pleased I was dating Jim also, as he didn't want me to be alone.

Life being life, new stones unexpectedly appeared in the path. Walking around them could not be avoided.

When I woke up one Sunday morning, Katie was lying beside my bed and not on her pad. I thought it a bit odd that she didn't move as I got ready for church. Jim met me there for the service, but when we returned, Katie was still there in the same spot, unable to get up on her own. We took her immediately to the emergency vet.

Congestive heart failure was the diagnosis. A decision had to be made, but it was not mine. Katie was Luke's dog. The vet told us she could last a day or two more and die naturally but perhaps painfully. We called Luke.

He took the news hard but said quietly, "She does not need to be in pain for a few more days on this earth. Katie has been so faithful and good to us all. Be kind and merciful to my girl, Mom. Set her free." He then asked me to put the phone to her ear so he could say goodbye one last time. Even with Luke in LA, we all held her close as she took her final breath.

Losing Katie was Luke's first significant heartbreak that month. Still, because of the strength of his AA brotherhood, he had the support he desperately needed to deal with emotional pain without reaching out for a substance. It was a major turning point for him. He now understood the power of the community and the strength that can come from actually living out the Serenity Prayer.

Luke's second test came right on the heels of Katie's passing. I was leaving choir rehearsal the following Wednesday evening when I got an odd text message from a number I did not recognize. It read, "Susan Paschal, I will love you for the rest of my life. Please forgive me."

"Who is this?" I texted back.

Ding. "Baxter. I am using a nurse's phone. I'm in the hospital. My kidneys have failed. Please come."

Baxter and I had officially been divorced for seven years, yet I felt compelled to go for Luke's sake. I called Jim to explain the situation, and he agreed to meet me at the hospital.

Worth, Luke's eldest brother, was there waiting for me. Baxter's kidneys were bleeding out, and he'd had a mild heart attack. The prognosis did not look good. The doctors would wait to start dialysis to see if kidney function returned, but it did not appear hopeful. Perhaps a kidney transplant was possible, but it would take months to figure out if he would be eligible or if/when one would be available.

I called Luke and gently broke the news that his father was hospitalized with possible kidney failure.

"There is no immediate danger, Bug. We'll just have to wait and see, so there is no need to panic," I cautiously told Luke, knowing the news would bring about a range of emotions.

Luke had been vacillating between love and hatred toward his

Chapter 5. The Circle of Life

father because of the divorce. Besides that, Luke's humiliation at his dad's incarceration and choosing an airplane over a house for us all left him feeling betrayed and abandoned. There was a lot of healing that needed to be done.

Luke took the news hard but again had deep support from his brotherhood, many of whom had had similar relationships with their fathers.

One way to encourage a possibility of healing Luke's pain would be if I made peace with Baxter and encouraged him to reach out to his son, asking for forgiveness. That was a tough order, but I knew I had to set an example, and that meant I needed to make peace to find true forgiveness in my heart for the man. After all, when anger remains in one's heart toward another human being, keeping it active is like drinking rat poison and expecting the rat to die.

*****

Later that fall, Jim and I flew down to spend Thanksgiving with my mother in Naples. I was a little nervous about how the meeting would go. One never knew what would come out of her mouth. She did not disappoint.

"Hello, Dr. Bartz, nice to meet you," Jim said politely when we walked in the door.

Her hands were on her hips, and the first words out of her mouth were "Where have you been hiding? I've only been praying for you for nine years!"

Before I could intervene to divert the conversation, Jim smiled and leaned his 6'3" frame down to hug her frail 5'1" body. She then blissfully led him away to show off the house, leaving me in the dust.

Jim immediately took on the role of her new "gopher" with loving enthusiasm. The next three days, he pulled down Christmas boxes from the attic, listened endlessly to her stories, did mail runs, and ensured she had enough paper towels and toilet paper to last a lifetime. By the end of our visit, Jim had totally won Mom over, as well as me.

Now on to Christmas! Luke had begun classes at the community college in Santa Monica that fall term and was making good grades. Sobriety and the 12 Step AA program were turning him into a man. Because of his good behavior, Luke was given a one-week reprieve to come home. I flew him and Jenni to North Carolina to meet Jim. My mother was too weak to travel, so at the Christmas candlelight service, Luke held up his phone in the church's darkness so she could hear me sing "O Holy Night" one last time. On Christmas morning, Jenni, Luke, and I would head down to Naples without Jim as he had to work the following day.

Upon our arrival, Mom was weak but had unique presents for all of us. Personal ones. Presents to remember her last Christmas with her family. We opened them quietly and took in the holiness of the occasion.

Later that evening, Luke told Grandma about Step Eight: Make a list of all the persons he had harmed and be willing to make amends to them all. Next to me, Luke felt he needed to make the most amends to her but tearfully told her he didn't know how. She absolved him with her usual talk of God's grace and her undying love and commitment to him. Mom gave a special gift to Luke that Christmas. She presented him with a ceramic angel and a promise that she'd never leave him, even after she passed away.

"I'll always be there for you, my boy. Remember, the veil is thin, and my love for you is strong. Keep up the good work. I am very proud of you," she whispered in his ear.

"I know, Grandma. The veil is thin indeed; remember, I've been there. I know you will be there for me. I will never forget all you have done for me. I love you so much. I'll make it. I promise," he told her with tears welling up in his eyes.

They said goodbye in a private moment the following day. I could see their hearts breaking when I took Luke to the airport, knowing this might be the last time they would see each other.

Jenni left the next day, and on December 31, I headed home to Jim. I treasured the memories and knew a good future lay ahead. This was the last Christmas with my mother. We both knew but never outwardly addressed that fact. We had a lifetime of Christmases and holy nights together to help me carry on.

In January, I moved into Jim's large home on a lake with Mom's blessing. We talked about marriage, but no final proposal was on the table. He promised it was coming, and I knew I had found my life partner deep in my heart. As the months flew by without drama, I could

Chapter 5. The Circle of Life

finally breathe as Mom was holding her own, or so it seemed from our daily chats.

Luke's graduation day was fast approaching at the end of June. Maybe he and Grandma could have one more visit. My mother however, was declining, and she decided she could no longer live alone. Jim had made it abundantly clear she was welcome to move in and take over the second floor, complete with her own suite and office. Plans were quickly put in place to tie up loose ends. I drove down to help her pack her belongings, and we made one final stop at her attorney's office. At the end of that meeting, I was given durable power of attorney over all her affairs.

I started the 12-hour trip back to Jim's house early on Thursday morning. The hours went by very fast. My mother talked the entire time, recalling her life, from stories of all her seven siblings, her courtship with my father, her starting her Shaklee business, and her last 21 glorious years with Joe. How I wish I had recorded it all.

That evening we had a nice dinner out on the back patio, talking excitedly about how Luke would be home five days after graduating from the sobriety house. We planned our graduation celebration for him, so proud that he finished the program. It had been a long day, and I was exhausted. Jim cleaned up the dishes before bed. My mother stayed outside for a long while, enjoying the fountain in the lake and the serenity of the evening. The sound of the crickets lulled me into a peaceful sleep.

Early the next morning, Jim and I took the dogs for a long walk. Before we left, I checked in on my mother She was sitting up in bed and said with the most glorious smile on her face, "Oh Susi, I know I will like it here." However, when we returned from our walk, Mom was sitting at the bottom of the staircase. With great calm, she told us that she had fallen down the steps and had broken her back and hip.

"God's calling me home, Susi! Call hospice," she said as I kicked into my numb mode.

It took a few hours to get all the players in place. Social workers came to assess her situation and then brought in a doctor for his approval. After her examination, we were advised a hip replacement would be in order, but after seeing the extent of her cancer, the doctor gave her the option to go back into hospice care and die at home.

Mom chose hospice without question. She was ready to go meet Jesus.

After looking at all her paperwork, the doctor said, "Ma'am, after reviewing these documents, I see the decision is not yours to make. You have given power of attorney to your daughter. It is her decision." The room fell silent. Looking at me, Mom cried out, reaching for my hand. "Susi, you promised to honor my wishes!"

How could I deny her request? She had given me life and had been my greatest love and support. Even though I did not want to say goodbye to my mother, I took her hand and told the doctor to call hospice. Quietly, Mom slipped off her rings and put them in my hand with a loving "Thank you, honey." My heart was breaking as I knew her time was coming quickly to an end.

While hospice was on its way, Mom asked for her phone to call her sisters and friends to say goodbye. No morphine until all calls were complete. It's a lovely experience to have a wake when the person is still alive.

My mother's last call was to Luke. He so wanted to get on an airplane that night to say goodbye in person, but she would not have it. She didn't want him to see her die. He understood. "I'll always be your angel" were her final words to him.

My mother's bed was set up facing the garden, and instructions were given regarding the morphine. She was not in pain except when Jim carefully picked her up to go to the bathroom when needed. Finally, we used diapers as she was fading fast and asking for more morphine drops.

Panic started setting in that I was giving her too much. Thank heavens, I had my personal doctor on call and reached out to Rebecca.

"I know Mom's dying, but I am afraid I will be the one to kill her with a morphine overdose!" I wailed into the phone.

"Tell me what the dosage is on the bottle, Susan, and tell me how much you are giving her," came her calm reply.

After I transmitted the information, Rebecca simply stated, "That's not enough to put down a chipmunk, my friend. It's her time, Susan. You are only easing her path home. I'm here for you. Give your mom a kiss for me." Relieved, I hung up and settled in for the long haul.

It was now Sunday morning. Neither Jim nor I had showered since

Chapter 5. The Circle of Life

Friday. We sat at the kitchen table, taking a break when he dropped to his knees.

"Susan, will you do me the honor of becoming my wife?" he asked lovingly.

"I'm a wreck, smelly and exhausted," I blurted out apologetically.

"Don't care," he said without moving.

With tears streaming down my face, I reached out for his welcoming arms, exclaiming, "Yes, I would love to marry you."

Jim responded, handing me a tissue, "I was planning a nice romantic evening for next week. My mother's ring is in the mail from my sister and has not yet arrived. I figured your mother would want to know my intentions before she passed."

Quietly we went in to see my mother, who was coming out of a deep sleep. Jim leaned over as she blinked her baby blues at him. "May I have your daughter's hand in marriage?" he asked, flirting back.

My mother smiled and nodded. "Now I can die in peace. Take care of my girl," she responded, patting his hand. She then gave us an Old Testament marriage blessing: "May the Lord of heaven prosper you both. May He grant you mercy and peace." She then closed her eyes and drifted off to sleep. Those were her last words to me as she never regained consciousness.

The days dragged on with the clanking oxygen machine keeping time like an old clock. My mother's Jesus music played in the background, just as she wanted. I slept on the sofa beside her every night until Wednesday evening when the death rattle started. It was too much to take in, so I went to bed upstairs. At 3 a.m., I was awakened by what seemed to be a kiss on my forehead. I jumped out of bed and ran downstairs, calling Jim's name.

Mom was no longer breathing but still very warm. Both Jim and I held her hands as her body cooled, thanking her for her life of service to others. It was a holy moment. No need to call hospice until daybreak, so we took a long, silent walk with the dogs under the stars.

Hospice came at 10 a.m., followed by the coroner. I walked with her body to the front door just as she had done for my father and Joe. Before they zipped up the burgundy velvet bag, I placed three pink roses from the garden in her hand. "'Well done, thou good and faithful servant.' I love you, Momma. Thank you for a lifetime of wonderful."

It was time to call Luke. Much to my surprise, he knew. He said he felt a kiss on his forehead at midnight Pacific time and knew it was Grandma. His bags were packed, and he was ready to come home. Graduation had taken place the night before. We were to pick him up at 9 that night in Fayetteville and start a new chapter in our lives.

Chapter 6

A New Start

"Every new beginning comes from some other beginning's end."—Seneca

My mother's service was uplifting and a beautiful tribute to her life. We all gathered at St. Peter, Daddy's old church in Arlington Heights, to say our final goodbyes. She was now at peace and was laid to rest next to my father. It was now time for us to go on with our lives.

As much as I had missed Luke, we both knew it was not a good idea for him to move back home. One tool taught in recovery to avoid relapse is having "new play toys, new playmates, and new playgrounds." North Carolina, therefore, was not an option as it would only be a familiar trigger for cravings.

Looking to continue his education, Luke applied to Kansas State for the fall and was accepted before leaving California. His grades had been very good at the community college in Santa Monica, which surprised me because his memory was still problematic. I encouraged him to stay in LA, which had more than 1500 AA meetings daily and a robust support system. But he wanted a real college experience and promised to find AA meetings on campus and stick to his sobriety program. Against my better judgment, I agreed and took out another student loan.

As an academic, I wanted Luke to have a good education. As a mother, I wanted to visit him on a big campus for parents' weekend, football games, and all the other fun aspects of college life. Luke left at the end of August. In short order, he called to tell me he had been rushed for a fraternity. My heart sank. One reason I have bad knees is that I spent a great deal of time kneeling on them in prayer.

Jim and I flew to Kansas for parents' weekend in October. Luke seemed to be doing well. He told me he was going to AA meetings. My gut told me he was drinking. Alcohol lessens inhibitions and can make someone in recovery think, "I drank, and I'm okay." This thought process can trigger a relapse. It did.

How stupid was I to think he could resist frat parties? By the semester's end, he was back to using drugs. I blamed myself. If I had not paid tuition, he could not have gone. Once again, I enabled him. *When will I learn?*

Luke came back home depressed and detoxing hard. He spent the first few weeks in his dark room sleeping and shaking while I was working through my rage at both of us. Again, putting my wants for Luke before my better judgment had to stop! I felt nauseated that I had taken out $35,000 in student loans with nothing to show for it but disaster. I suppose "live and learn" is a part of everyone's journey, but my lack of courage and inability to trust my instincts had devastating consequences. To quote Forrest Gump, "Stupid is as stupid does."

Luke begged to return to Kansas State in January, promising to leave the frat and find a sober roommate. *No. Not an option. Not this time.* I finally got the message that my enabling behavior would take us both down. Luke was an adult and therefore in charge of making his own decisions, but I held the purse strings, and they were drawn shut.

I was still in the early stages of understanding that addiction was a disease and needed to be treated as such. I had yet to learn that relapse was common in early sobriety and that SUD is a complex disease requiring physical, mental, and spiritual treatment. People with SUD have distorted thinking and thus distorted behaviors. Luke did not lose his sobriety to chemical cravings this time; his receptors had been tamed for more than a year. He lost it to his need to fit in and be normal, an issue he would have to sort out for himself.

The Christmas season was a somber one for all of us. Jim tended to the dogs, and I kept to myself, going on long walks grieving my stupidity, Luke's failings, and my mother's absence.

After three weeks of living in relative solitude, I heard him sobbing in the shower. He had hit bottom. The bottom is the place that most people with drug and alcohol dependency can reach before they are finally ready to admit they have a problem and reach out for help. *Dang, I had thought he had already been there, but then I realized*

Chapter 6. A New Start

he could always count on me to bail him out. When would I hit my bottom?

When Luke came downstairs, he was clean shaven and calm.

"I take full responsibility for my actions, Mom," he said with remorse.

I simply nodded, not quite able to engage.

He continued, "I can't take this insane dance anymore and am willing to do whatever it takes to maintain my sobriety. I need to rework my steps and have been rereading the Big Book and talking to my old sponsor. Deep inside, I guess I had hoped I could be like other men. I see now I can't and never will."

Again, I just nodded.

He apologized to Jim and me for his lack of judgment, telling us he was going to a sobriety house in the mountains of North Carolina. He couldn't face going back to LA as a failure and wanted to get back on his program closer to home, at least for the time being. He felt he could get back on his feet in three months and had already called the house. They had a slot for him with insurance coverage approval.

"I've used the money Grandma left me for the co-pay. I've cost you too much already," he said, lowering his eyes.

Finally, I was ready to respond. "I forgive you, Luke. I've made a lot of mistakes in my life too. This time, however, I will let you pay the tab." He agreed without hesitation.

Jim drove Luke to the mountains in Asheville two days later while I stayed home and cried.

*****

January 2013 was unusually cold and gloomy for North Carolina. So was I. Grieving the loss of my mother, planning a wedding, teaching full-time, and running a business I knew little about kept me running fast in a numb, bipolar state of mind. Every moment I could feel the boulder of expectations and fear careening behind me, ready to run me over. One day at a time. One project at a time.

With Luke safe in the sobriety house, at least I was free from worrying about him. Jim and I had set a date for our wedding, May 4, two days after my last day of teaching. I wish I had thought that one through better, but it looked doable on paper.

It was time to look for a wedding dress. I had seen some lovely pictures online, but to be totally honest, I had not given the dress much thought. I just wanted to run away to the beach with a bottle of champagne with a few good friends. Jim, however, never had a real wedding before. A justice of the peace conducted his first wedding ceremony before Jim had left for his tour in Germany. He wanted a more formal affair this time, and I lovingly obliged.

On my way home from school one day, I pulled into the parking lot of a bridal salon. It was sleeting and dismal outside, which matched my mood. But I knew I had to get a dress sooner or later, so I went in looking much like a drowned rat.

"How can I help you today?" asked the young assistant as I walked in the door.

I'm sure she thought I was the mother or grandmother of the bride as her jaw dropped when I told her I had come to look at wedding dresses for myself. Quickly on the rebound, she hustled me into a stall with 101 questions about style, date, and venue. Much to her chagrin, my response was simply "I haven't a clue."

She must have seen Mom's Jaguar parked out front as she dug in with abandon, intent on selling me her finest. "We have some stunning dresses I know will be perfect for you!"

"No, no—nothing fancy. Been there, done that," I said, seeing the glint in her eye. She had no ears.

"Oh, honey, with your figure, I can see a mermaid or trumpet style..."

"Whatever," I muttered from a state of blah.

She waltzed in with three blingy, strapless white wedding dresses. In my mind's eye, visions of myself when "the girls" were still above my navel without a hoist blinded reality. I conceded to try on her picks. She grinned boldly when I stepped into the first mermaid gown.

"Oh, darlin'—you still got it! You look stunning!" she yapped as she zipped up the dress. With minimal hope, I turned around to face the full-length mirror.

That's when it hit. I stood stunned for five seconds taking in the image before letting out a gargantuan hoot that rocked the saleslady back 10 feet. There in front of me stood the warrior queen of hospitals, rehabs, and hospice pimped up in a white froufrou dress. *No, I need to be in red or black velvet with flaming torches shooting out of my arms and a firearm strapped to my side.* The vision was so comical I sat down and started laughing uncontrollably. She didn't know quite how to react. I thanked her and left. At least I had a good chuckle that day. Thankfully Caryl, Reggie, and Jeannette came over one day and whisked me off to another bridal shop, where they picked out a beautiful, age-appropriate gown for me.

*****

The weeks raced as I struggled to plan for our upcoming wedding in May. My spirits were lifted to hear Luke was making a remarkable transition. The sobriety house had its own gym where he spent hours each day working out along with going to meetings. He took great pride in the fact that he quickly became a role model and was looked up to by all, leading many of the group discussions and sharing his experiences. Even the counselors were learning Luke's new techniques from his previous program.

At home, I was starting to research SUD and found that regular exercise in addiction recovery can help prevent a return to alcohol or drug use by as much as 95 percent.[1] These studies also found that exercise can help manage stress, depression, and anxiety, which can all contribute to substance use. Luke needed all these things to keep sober from a neurobiological perspective. So much of SUD, especially dual diagnosis, is about balancing brain chemistry, not just behavior modification and learning to walk a spiritual path of surrender. It was eye-opening to realize that

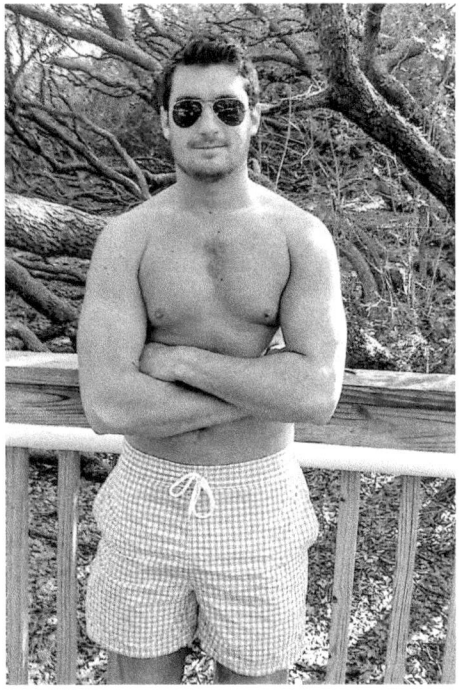

This is what healthy 21-year-old Luke looked like after the second rehab.

exercise releases endorphins to the body, creating a natural high. These feelings are similar to the endorphins people experience when abusing substances.

In April, Luke came home from the sobriety house. Gone was the terrified boy that left in January. In front of me stood a confident, well-built man filled with hope and resolve. He had decided in the mountains that it would be in his best interest to return to his AA brotherhood in LA, look for a job to support himself and try to break into acting. As much as I wanted him closer, in my heart, I knew it was the right decision. I agreed to help him with rent and expenditures until he got on his feet as long as he stayed clean. He had secured a roommate from the sobriety house in the mountains and an apartment. Eventually, he wanted to return to school, but for now, he needed to prove that he could maintain his sobriety while living independently.

On May 4, Luke walked me down the aisle. It was a special ceremony for my family and everyone attending, as it brought hope for all. Many people in our church had been there with Luke and me throughout all the tragedies, as Jim's friends had been there for him through his heartbreaking divorce. It was then I saw the wisdom of Jim wanting a large wedding. It was not only for us to enjoy but for everyone to celebrate as a community, giving us a chance to thank each one for their unfailing support.

Instead of the traditional father/daughter first dance, Luke and I had a son/mother dance. We had many special moments reaffirming our bond to always be a team. Adding Jim was not a threat. My family was now complete. Indeed, the sun had come out after the storm.

Jim and I postponed our honeymoon until October. I was simply too exhausted to go right after the wedding. And we needed to launch Luke and set him up to live in Los Angeles.

We put him on an airplane three days later. Back in California, Luke dove in and got settled in his new place. His friends were supportive and welcomed him back into the AA fold. He was not the first or the last to have a relapse only to rebound bigger and better. He was, as he wrote in a post, "Back in the game."

We agreed Luke would only have sober roommates—my stipulation for paying the rent. However, his friend from the mountains went

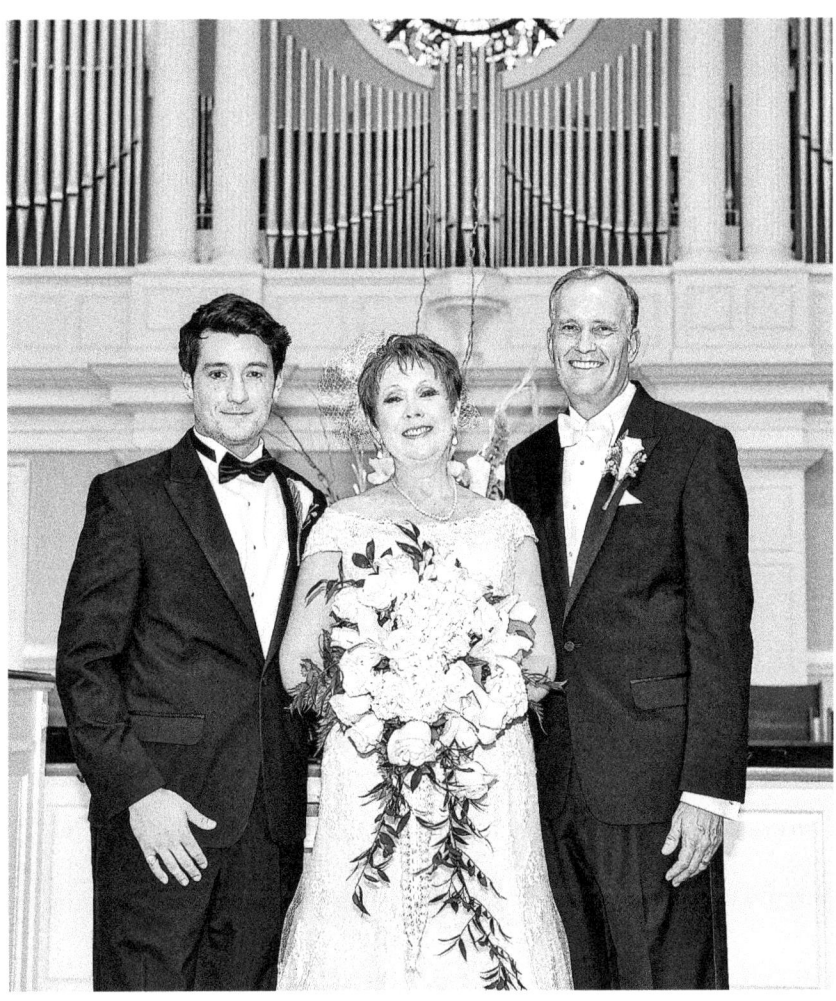

Luke, me, and Jim on May 3, 2013.

back home after only three months. LA was too foreign for him as he was a country boy at heart, leaving his father and me to sort out the lease and other bills by phone. With great rage, the father told me he'd rather have a son with cancer than one who was an addict.

I was appalled that a father could make such a statement about his child! Did he not know addiction was a disease? I wish I had known about the film *Stop the Shame: Addicts Hear Comments Cancer Patients Never Would* back then, as I would have sent him the link along with our half of the electric bill.[2] Pat Matuszak of Cumberland Hall Hospital in Hopkinsville, Kentucky, wrote a heart-wrenching summary on the hospital's website:

> A teenage boy lies in a hospital bed with IV tubes attached to his arm. His scalp and eyebrows are missing hair—signs of chemotherapy. He looks worried as he focuses his eyes from one of his frowning parents to the other, then drops his gaze as if expecting trouble. His parents take turns launching angry questions and accusations. It becomes clear that they are blaming him for having cancer: Why did he let this happen? Why is he putting them through this? Why doesn't he just decide to get up and be well?
>
> Anyone viewing this interaction would be stunned. Who would ever be so cruel to treat their child this way when he is going through a devastating illness? The scene pauses, and words scroll across the screen: What if we treated people with cancer the way we treat people with addiction? Addiction is a disease.

Wouldn't it be nice if parents, society, and especially the medical community all treated people with addiction the way we treat people with cancer? But they didn't know. It would take until October 2019 for the American Society of Addiction Medicine to release a new definition of addiction.[3] It reads as follows:

> Addiction is a treatable, chronic medical disease involving complex interactions among the brain circuits, genetics, the environment, and an individual's life experiences. People with addiction use substances or engage in behaviors that become compulsive and often continue despite harmful consequences. Prevention efforts and treatment approaches for addiction are generally as successful as those for other chronic diseases.

In 2013 we were all still living in a world ruled by Stigma.

Luke quickly found another roommate, but in short order, the new one started using drugs again. I was proud of Luke for telling him he had to leave without my prompting. It was a stretch to pay full rent at LA prices, but one I was willing to take on to keep him safe.

After a few weeks, Luke started taking acting classes, where he met Jacob, a man who would become one of his best friends for life. Jacob was not in recovery but was well-grounded and supportive of Luke's sobriety. They did not live together but instantly became constant companions.

Jacob and Luke were both Hollywood handsome. One evening while dining out, they were both approached to be on the TV program *The Bachelor*. Both ended up turning the offer down. Jacob

Chapter 6. A New Start

feared being on the program might hinder his serious quest to become a successful film actor. Luke turned it down because he suspected they wanted to focus on his recovery story. For Luke, that was a very private and spiritual matter. He would not let anyone pollute it commercially.

Soon Luke was getting minor roles in student films from USC and in a TV commercial. While Jim and I were on our honeymoon, Luke called to tell me about some challenges he faced breaking into show business. I laughed. "Welcome to the world of acting, son." We could talk about this topic for hours as it was once my profession too.

"Son, it's just the way of 'the Biz,'" I reminded him.

From his voice, I could tell he was sober and happy, finding the strength to go out and feel comfortable in his own skin. I kept looking for signs of weakness but found none. That is not to say I didn't worry. That is the way of "The Mother."

Luke came home for Christmas, a delight for me but painful for him as his father quickly lost ground. Baxter and his sons spent quality time together over the holidays. I was more than dismayed to learn they all had been drinking in front of Luke. Luke said he didn't mind and told me he often went out with some friends who drank. Out of respect for Luke, Jim and I tried never to have any wine or beer in front of him. But Luke was right; if he was to learn to live in the world sober, he would need to stay the course no matter what others did.

*****

In late January 2014, I received a call from Baxter's son Worth. Baxter had a heart attack and was in surgery. A quadruple bypass was needed, then a pacemaker. Without pause, I booked Luke a flight home to see his dad. Even though the doctors felt confident Baxter had more time, I wanted Luke to have a chance to say goodbye just in case he didn't. On this trip home, Luke started to complain about his back hurting. I could tell he wasn't drug-seeking, just stating a fact that would prove crucial the following year.

In the days before Luke arrived, I spent time with Baxter, telling him again how important it was to make sure Luke knew how much he loved him and was proud of him. No matter what Momma said, he also needed to hear that confirmation from his father. Me, always meddling.

But from experience, Baxter always required some prodding as personal conversations were uncomfortable.

Not this time. I was pleasantly surprised when Baxter told me they had been calling and texting regularly and creating a new healthy bond. Both promised that would continue for whatever time Baxter had left. Even though the goodbye was tear-filled for both, Luke told me they were at peace with each other. Love overcame the pains of the past. Such is the power of forgiveness.

Ever since the accident, the month of February had been difficult. Where it had once been a month of joy celebrating Luke's birthday, it had turned into a time of trying to process the trauma after his accident. I was looking for my "new normal," as nurse Patty had predicted.

The first anniversary of the accident was a blur. My body seemed to remember, and every time I passed a cross on the side of the highway, I would start to shake with the words *I almost lost him, I almost lost him!* screaming through my head.

The second year I was still numb, unable to feel much of anything. For the past 10 years, I had dealt with losses, cancers, deaths, and a near-death tragedy, leaving my heart frozen. My saving grace was a beautiful text that day from Luke.

On the third anniversary of the accident, the bottom dropped out for me. Jim had left for work, and I'd plopped down to read and journal in my chair. Something in me snapped when the date came up on my computer, February 6. I started to shake uncontrollably and weep. Those tears quickly evolved

---

Date: Mon, 6 Feb 2012 23:01:33 -
From: lukepaschal@gmail.com
To: susanbpaschal@hotmail.com

arent you glad i'm alive?
2 years ago today I faced the eyes of whoever is out there. They held me for a brief moment only to materialize into what we perceive it as "no... I still need him to do something, he's not ready". Only through that beaten and battered state was I able to see the nature of true beauty and understanding of all things around me. Yet I was clouded by my own selfish behavior and alcoholism. Mother I love you and thank you so much for these past 2 years putting up with my bullshit. I can't wait to spend the next 30 making it up to you.

Luke's second-year reflection on his NDE.

Chapter 6. A New Start

into nausea, shaking, and screaming. It went on for more than an hour. *I almost lost him, I almost lost him!* repeated over and over in my brain, along with the simple word *Momma*...

Everything I was experiencing was called PTSD.[4] Mayo Clinic website describes post-traumatic stress disorder as developing in people who have experienced shocking, scary, or dangerous events. Fear triggers split-second changes, helping the body defend against danger.

My body had finally decided it was time I could start feeling again. Although the release was traumatic, it was also freeing—to a point. I would always worry about Luke, but at least my cry of *I almost lost him, I almost lost him!* turned into *I almost lost him, but I didn't*.

At the fourth anniversary, I worried about Luke facing his PTSD with the added burden of another crisis looming on his horizon: losing his father. *Would he be strong enough to face this pain?* I could only hope and pray.

All in all, 2014 held promise. Luke returned to LA after seeing his father and focused on his new career and sobriety. He felt confident going back in the game. His face looked much better, showing only minimal scarring after plastic surgery to fix the gashes left by the accident.

In retrospect, I was apprehensive about his surgery at first, but my girlfriend Rebecca volunteered to be his anesthesiologist and took over his pain management. Rebecca assured me she could pick out the best drugs that would not cause a neurobiological reaction that might cause cravings.[5] Fingers crossed. Over-the-counter Advil and topical non-narcotic pain sprays would be administered for aftercare. No narcotics would be used. She also told me his tolerance for the anesthesia had been very high and that he fought losing consciousness—information I would need to remember in the future.

At Thanksgiving, we had a professional photographer take a family portrait. Jim would never replace Baxter, but he gave Luke grounding and a feeling of security. Luke never called Jim dad, but he did introduce us to others as his parents with great pride.

Back in LA, Luke was putting himself out there, pounding the pavement looking for work. Acting is not the best way to make money—breaking into "the biz" is difficult and costs more than one makes starting out, even after one gets moderately successful. I was willing

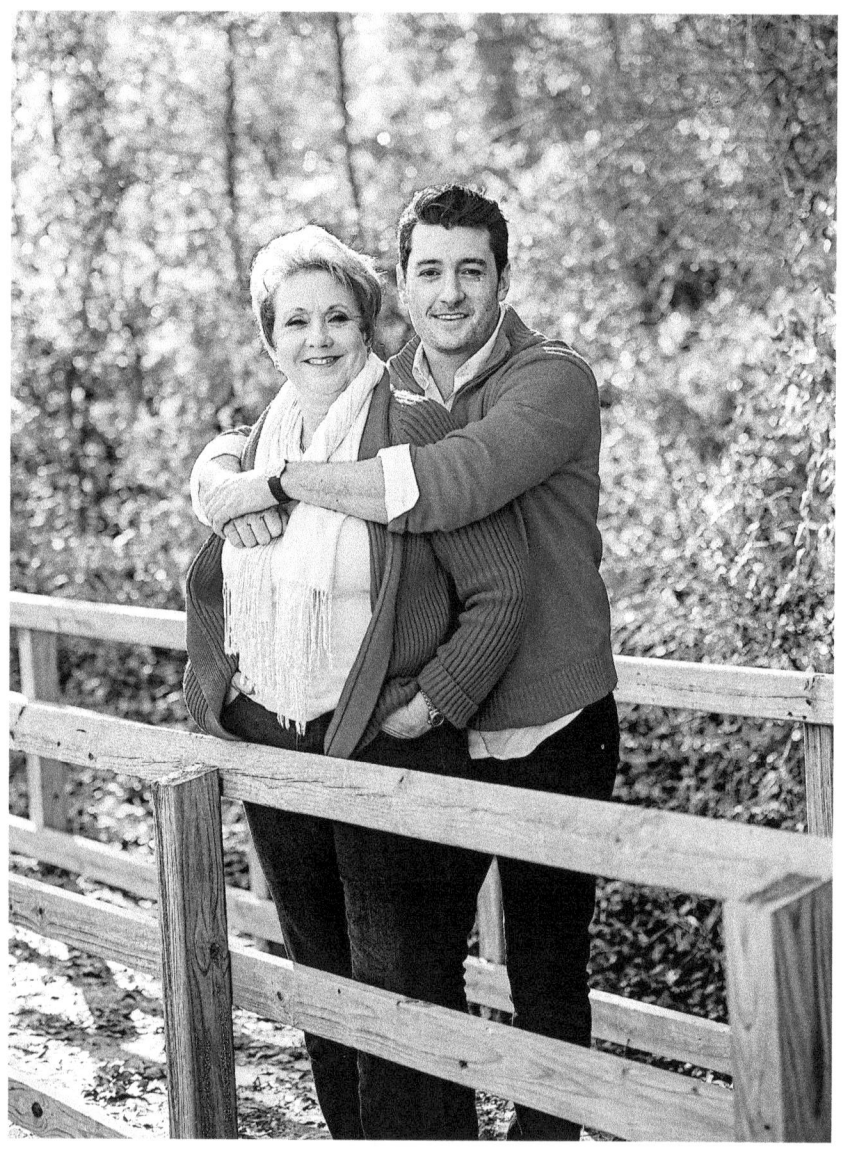

Susan and Luke, November 2014.

to take on the extra costs because I knew pursuing this avenue was building his confidence and giving him time to attend AA meetings daily.

The hustle and bustle of LA was exciting for Luke, which was a good thing. It kept his endorphins kicking in high gear. Luke was a

Chapter 6. A New Start

natural on camera and had been cast in a few short films, giving him more professional credits toward a SAG-AFTRA professional actors union card.

He also secured a job as a driver for a foreign car company that provided a cab-like service for a high-end hotel in Santa Monica. His job was to deliver a three-minute spiel about the car to the occupants and then drop them off at their local destination. He loved it. He loved cars and talking about them. The job helped him learn about the city and put extra cash in his pocket. Unfortunately, the job soon ended when the car company's contract expired.

Luke was a sensitive soul like me and felt terrible that I still supported him. I could also tell the natural grind of seeking employment as an actor was discouraging as he was tired of pounding the pavement for acting jobs—a discouragement I more than understood. Luke and I texted daily, but he usually only called when he had great news to share or needed something. I never knew what to expect. One day in late May, he called.

"Hey, Mom! I went out today and put in six applications to some high-end fashion boutiques on Rodeo Drive in Beverly Hills. They liked me, especially one guy at Etro, the Italian fashion house," Luke excitedly reported.

Pause…. Long pause. "Son, you do realize some people work more than 10 years in retail trying to advance themselves enough to secure a fashion apprenticeship at stores on Rodeo Drive? You have no retail experience. Nada," I cautioned.

"I know, but they liked me!" he spouted back.

I told him not to get his hopes up and keep looking around. Maybe start off at the lower-end stores. Hotels. Restaurants, perhaps—the choice job for unemployed actors. He was undeterred. Three weeks later, I got another call.

"Hey, Mom, Etro hired me with a good salary and benefits! I start on Monday, and guess what? They give me two suits, shirts, and shoes to wear! Etro suits and I can keep them all. Hopefully, I can earn enough to put some aside and still attend after-hours auditions."

Luke was elated, and I was dumbfounded but not too surprised. He was a born salesman who often talked his way into getting goodies from family and friends. His father always remarked that Luke

Luke Paschal
August 8, 2014

New fresh clothes, brought to you by ETRO. #newsuits #suitup #matchingshoes #milan #rodeo #lovemywork #freeeeeeee

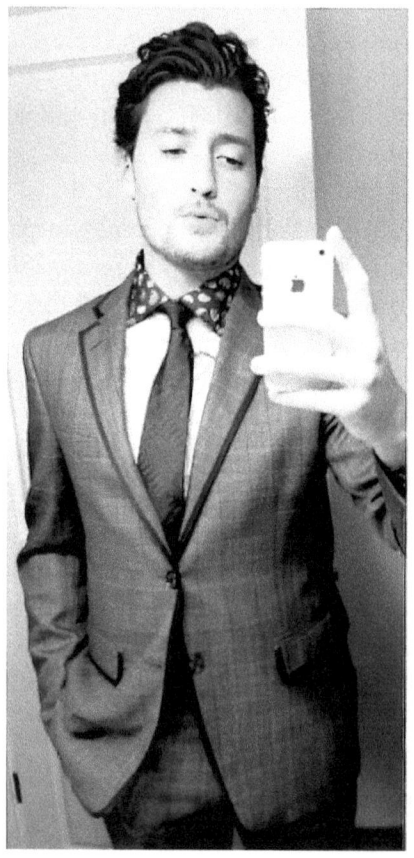
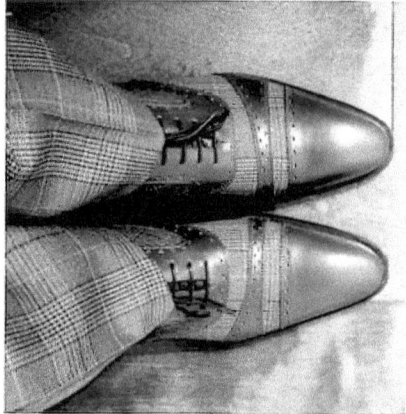
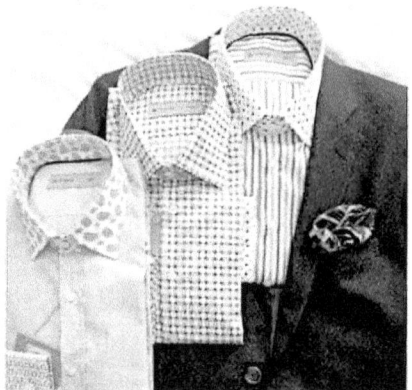

Luke in his new Etro wardrobe.

could sell ice to an Eskimo in Alaska during a blizzard. Luke indeed had an engaging personality and was a fashionista at heart. Ever since he was a boy, I knew that shopping with a daughter would pale in comparison to shopping with him. For hours Luke would hunt out precisely what he wanted—designer, of course—and wore clothes like a model.

"Good job, Bug. Good job," I said with pride.

Chapter 6. A New Start

"Told you so, Momma," he said in his *I told you so* tone of voice. Dang!

*****

In the meantime, Baxter was losing ground. I took my turn driving him to Pinehurst for appointments a few times, always going out to lunch afterward. He was doing dialysis every night, and I knew he was going stir-crazy at home and could use a fun outing. It also gave us time to say our goodbyes. I barely recognized the man. Sickness ages a person and brings opportunities for closure.

On our last outing, Baxter broke down in tears over lunch, something I thought I would never see. He told me how sorry he was for failing Luke and me. I could tell he had tried to make up for his lack of fathering by being there for his grandchildren. In tears, we held hands and reminisced about our good times together. That was the last day I ever saw him alive.

Thank heavens Luke had been at home to see him one last time. On July 19, I received a frantic call from Worth. Baxter had woken up feeling odd and knew he was in trouble. He drove himself to the nearest emergency room. No sooner had he hobbled in the door but he collapsed and coded. Baxter died shortly after Worth arrived at the hospital. Worth called Luke to break the news.

I wish I had told Luke, but I knew it was a good thing he heard it from his brother. Luke had been surfing with Jacob in Malibu when he got the call. Thank heavens Jacob was with Luke as he sobbed on the beach.

Etro gave Luke four days off to come home for the funeral. He was stoic but clearly got great comfort from being with his extended family.

The night after the funeral, I went home and cried not only for Luke but for the fact that a significant chapter of our life was truly over. Jim had to leave the funeral to attend a training session in Atlanta, and I was left alone with the dogs and my memories. All the anger I once felt for Baxter was gone, and I only felt compassion and sadness for what might have been. Our son was the one blessing of that union; I will always be grateful.

The next day I took Luke back to the airport. He was sad but sober, from what I could tell. I gave him a lot of credit for resisting everyone's urges to stay home for a while, but he knew he needed to get back to work. We both looked forward to seeing each other in California in just a few weeks for the upcoming Shaklee convention in Long Beach.

The convention lasted three days, leaving the rest of the week for play. One day we drove to Rodeo Drive to see Luke at work. I was truly impressed to see the boutique and even more impressed that he was folding the shirts for display. Perfect folds and creases. He'd never have another excuse for crumpling them up at home. It helped that Yarrow flew out to spend time with us. Though they were not romantically involved, they were cherished friends.

Luke seemed to have everything under control, but he kept complaining about back pain. I assumed it was a ploy for self-medicating. I didn't see if he was drinking or doing drugs, but maybe I didn't want to see it. There is a fine line to walk being a parent of a child with SUD. At 23, he was no longer a child and needed to take full responsibility for his disease.

The bottom fell out in October when Luke told us he had to quit Etro because of his back pain. He promised he was not doing drugs but told me his back hurt so bad being on his feet all day. Plus, he missed acting. The job did not allow any time for auditions. He asked to come home for a few weeks, and I agreed. Luke needed his family and time to grieve.

The upcoming year held a lot of promise. Luke returned to Los Angeles excitedly as he had booked a photo shoot to try his hand at modeling. An old saying is "What does not kill me makes me stronger."

 Luke Paschal
November 10, 2014

I ask you right here please to agree with me that a scar is never ugly. That is what the scar makers want us to think. But you and I, we must make an agreement to defy them. We must see all scars as beauty. Okay? This will be our secret. Because take it from me, a scar does not form on the dying. A scar means, I survived.

Luke's post reflecting on scars.

Nietzsche, I believe. Such was the case with my son. He was learning to take what scars life gave him and turn them into strengths. He never wanted to be cast as the pretty boy but rather as a character with grit, depth, and compassion; indeed, that was who he was becoming.

The fact was he was a pretty boy too. Hollywood handsome, my girlfriends called him. His modeling shoot portfolio landed him a few small jobs. In his spare time, from pounding the pavement to find work, he threw himself into personal development, working out for hours, going to two AA meetings a day, meditating, and learning how to build himself up nutritionally.

*****

With more spare time on my hands, I threw myself back into reading current literature on SUD. It never made sense to me that addicts were called "morally flawed" when they relapsed. Would you blame a cancer patient as morally deficient if their cancer returned? Cancer is, after all, up to 10 percent genetic.[6] The rest is caused by environmental and lifestyle choices.

My learning was hindered, however, as most of the SUD literature is written in medicalese and published in journals only professionals can access. Recovery centers try to break down the info, but who knows to look there, especially on your first go-round?

It was disheartening to find that brain recovery after addiction is complex. It takes someone with advanced training in addiction to unpack the information. After scouring the internet for years, I had yet to find a readable layman's explanation. What I could put together is that SUD is not a "one size fits all" disease. Like cancer, there are different levels of severity, and different drugs damage various parts of the brain. I prayed Luke's brain had not been so severely damaged that it could never recover. Few studies had been done, however, to give me answers.

Luckily, I found that research was being done by a few recovery specialists who noted that a healthy diet and good nutritional supplementation could help heal the brain after extended drug use.

One book in particular caught my attention, *End Your Addiction Now: The Proven Nutritional Supplement Program That Can Set You Free* by Dr. Charles Gant. Until then, Luke believed in nutrition but took it with a grain of salt since the ideas had come from Grandma and me. What did we know? Coming from leading experts—now he'd listen. What parent cannot relate? Gant's book put together a protocol for healing the brain using nutraceuticals and even broke down the different kinds of protocols for other drug cravings. We stocked up.

I also read up on the brain's ability to heal from the work of Dr. Daniel Amen, a pioneer in brain research.[7] The Amen clinics use a brain imaging diagnostic tool called SPECT (single photon emission computed tomography) that views the brain to help accurately identify underlying brain issues contributing to symptoms. I never thought about it before, but as Dr. Daniel Amen often points out, the brain is the only organ doctors treat without observing its function. Can you imagine a cardiologist treating a heart patient by only listening to his symptoms without ever getting an electrocardiogram or ultrasound? Or an orthopedic surgeon trying to set a bone without an x-ray? It made no sense.

What made even less sense was that there were virtually no monies or endowments to help find a cure due to the stigma surrounding the disease. According to an article in STAT News by Lev Fatcher, "Venture capital firms invested just $130 million into novel addiction treatments in the past 10 years, compared to a nearly $36 billion bet on oncology."[8] Maybe there would be more funding if the pharmaceutical companies offered more drug options like Suboxone. But they always look at the bottom line for profit. The stigma of addiction keeps people from asking for help. AA/NA does not publish recovery statistics. How could anyone know what, if any, treatment works?

Lack of funding also leaves medical schools in a bind. Dr. Timothy Brennan, director of the Addiction Institute at Mt. Sinai and St. Luke's in New York, was quoted in the *New York Times* article "Most Doctors Are Ill-Equipped to Deal with the Opioid Epidemic." He stated, "Combating the addiction crisis with our limited resources is like trying to fight World War II with only the Coast Guard."[9]

*****

Our annual Shaklee convention in 2015 was in Pleasanton, California. Lucky for us, it was in February, which coincided with Luke's 24th birthday, so Jacob and Luke drove up from Los Angeles to celebrate. We

Chapter 6. A New Start

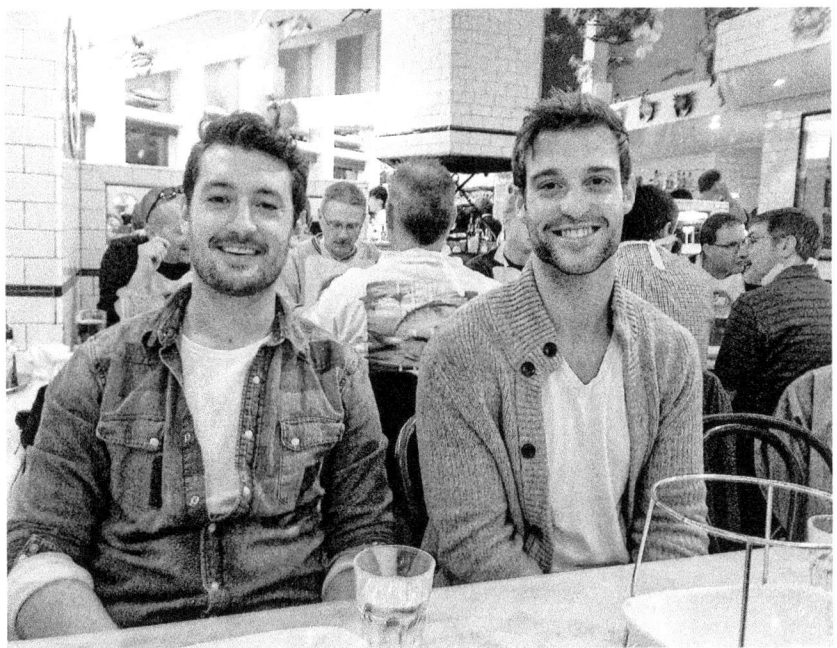

Luke's 24th birthday in San Francisco with his best friend, Jacob Taylor.

rode the trolley, went on sightseeing tours, and ate ourselves silly. Luke loved crab, so off we went to Fisherman's Wharf.

Drinking in front of Luke was not an option, but no one noticed. Luke would sit at a table and turn his wineglass upside down. The rest of us followed suit. To compensate for the waiter's look of disappointment, we'd order inordinate amounts of appetizers along with bottles of sparkling water. All went back home full and happy.

It was as if the universe knew what was coming and was giving us wonderful and quality time together to give us strength to face the life-changing challenges that would come in the summer.

Jim's sister lived in Oahu, Hawaii, so we decided to see her and then vacation in Maui. Luke came along. He meditated every morning, ending his workout with a run down the coast. We all went scuba diving, and Luke jumped off small cliffs into swirling waters below, scaring me silly. Seeing him so happy took the edge off of my fears. Boys. Some never grow out of shortening their mother's life with their antics.

On this trip, however, we were also given more signs that something was wrong with Luke's back. A long boat ride on the ocean took us careening over large waves, slamming us down after every crest. Jim and I were thrilled as we held tightly onto the ropes. Luke kept reaching for his lower back and grimacing. I could tell he was in real pain and not drug-seeking. *But why his lower back? The rods and screws were in his mid-back. Maybe it was referred pain?* I was concerned but respected his privacy.

We all returned to North Carolina as Luke was invited to speak at a Shaklee health and wellness seminar to tell his recovery story through lifestyle changes. Luke, indeed, was an entrepreneur and, as we soon found out, a gifted public speaker. He was captivating and thrilled to share the stage with Dr. Stephen Chaney, a celebrated professor from the University of North Carolina. I just sat back in awe and pride.

While he was home Luke and I talked about his acting endeavors. The trip to Maui woke Luke up to the fact that he didn't have the drive his friend Jacob had concerning acting as a profession. Luke realized he was meant to be an entrepreneur and immediately took a Tony Robbins business training seminar.

"I don't know how, Mom, but I'm going to build my own empire one day, just like Roger Barnett," he exclaimed on a weekly call when he got back to LA.

That endeavor would soon be put on hold. In late June, he called in tears. The pain in his lower back was excruciating. We already had x-rays of his upper back that showed nothing was out of place with his back apparatus. I suggested he go to UCLA and have a CT scan of his entire back. Something was clearly wrong.

Luke called the next day. "Mom—do I have an IVC filter?"

"What is that?" I asked, genuinely puzzled.

"I don't know, but the doctors asked me to find out," he replied.

I went to my church choir that night and asked a medical doctor friend of mine what an IVC filter looked like. He took out a marker and on a napkin drew a small sketch of what looked to be a metal spider, telling me it was used to prevent blood clots. The light bulb went on! I called Luke back immediately.

"Yes, son, you do have one. I completely forgot! It was threaded through a vein in your groin when you were in a coma right after your accident."

He replied with trepidation, "The doctors thought so, but it is not where it is supposed to be. It's migrated and is poking holes in my intestines and aorta. It also rubs up against my spinal column—thus the pain."

I was thrown back into full panic mode. "Pack your bags—you're coming home for an extended stay," I demanded.

Chapter 7

The Unseen Enemy

"Most people talk about fear of the unknown, but if there is anything to fear, it is the known."—Deepak Chopra

Luke stepped off the plane in North Carolina, frightened and in pain, ready to face the unknown. A local vascular surgeon examined Luke's CT scan. He told us Luke's case was far too complex for his skills. He promptly contacted an experienced vascular surgeon at Duke. Thankfully it was only an hour's drive from where we lived. We went home, awaiting a call to set up a consultation.

One night Luke and I watched TV together, trying to keep our minds off the inevitable removal of the filter. While surfing the channels, we stumbled across a news story about filter failures. We were stunned to learn multiple manufacturers were involved. Some filters had been known to migrate and break apart, injuring and even killing some unsuspecting people. We also learned that since Luke's accident, the FDA had required IVC filters to be used only as temporary fixes, not permanent solutions to prevent blood clots. Luke and I looked at each other in disbelief as we were led to believe it could stay in for the duration of his life.

"Mom, I could have gotten this thing taken out safely years ago?" Luke asked.

"That's my take, son," I replied, connecting the dots.

"You think maybe we should contact a lawyer?" he asked tentatively.

"Bug," I answered in dismay, "you just may have a medical malpractice lawsuit on your hands from what we saw tonight."

We sat in silence, stunned. I tried to hide my fear and rage. My son had already been through so much and now faced another surgery.

Chapter 7. The Unseen Enemy

This meant being put back on narcotics. *This surgery could have been avoided!* We would have been clueless if we had not seen that program on television. We immediately began looking for personal injury attorneys to take his case.

Days later, we met with Dr. Anderson at Duke University Medical Center. He was a kind, elderly physician who did removals daily. Though jovial upon our introduction, his demeanor turned grim as he studied Luke's CT scan.

Finally, he broke his silence. "This filter may be difficult to remove. At least five spikes are deeply embedded in the surrounding tissue. One is against your spine, and four others penetrate your colon and aorta."

Luke listened carefully, tight-lipped, as the doctor continued. "If you were an old man like me, I'd suggest leaving it in. But at your age and activity level, one wrong twist from a rigorous activity could cause the spike to rupture the aorta, resulting in an instant bleed out. The choice is yours, however."

I inhaled sharply, trying to maintain my composure as Dr. Anderson began sharing the details of the procedure. "I'll thread a wire through the jugular vein to hook the filter and remove it. This procedure works for most people. We'll pull it out with luck, and you can go home that day."

Luke glanced in my direction, looking hopeful, but I was worried. *I know there's a "but" coming,* I thought. There was.

"But," Dr. Anderson said, "if that doesn't work, we must choose option two, re-opening your abdominal cavity, cutting through your old scar. This could lead to intestinal blockages as new scarring can adhere to the intestines. If your aorta is compromised, we'll need to clamp off blood flow using a heart-lung bypass machine."

Good Lord, what am I hearing? I almost passed out. I knew enough about anatomy to understand that the vena cava and aorta are underneath all his organs in his chest cavity. After nearly losing Luke once, the thought of such a risky and invasive operation was almost too much for me to handle. Luke sat staring at the floor, and I went numb, back to that old safe place where feelings run and hide when matters get too frightening.

Before ending the appointment, the doctor told Luke if the first surgery did not work, they would wake him up and ask him again if he wanted to go on with the more invasive extraction. We both looked at Luke for his approval.

"Sounds like a plan," Luke replied with confidence. It made him feel good to know he would have the final say. With the surgery date set for three weeks, Luke would have enough time to consider his options. I knew he was the only one who could make that determination.

*****

When we got home, Luke was quiet, tired, and withdrawn. He feared the surgery, but his greatest fear was being put back on pain meds. He called his sponsor for support.

One week later, Luke and I met with the physician's assistant to discuss Luke's medical history and for a physical exam. Luke wanted to speak with the PA alone, but I insisted on being in the room for the medical history portion. Not only did I know more about his original injuries, but I also wanted to make sure the PA knew the extent of Luke's chemical dependence and request a substance abuse consult to manage his meds. I told myself I trusted Luke. I didn't. I knew he would be ashamed and embarrassed.

Unfortunately, because of the stigma associated with addiction, many people afflicted with SUD will not be honest with their doctors. A 2020 study by Dr. Brandon Muncan et al. states, "Healthcare providers—even well-meaning ones—who do not acknowledge that disclosure of a patient's substance use history can have catastrophic consequences for that patient are not serving their patient's best interests or adhering to the principle of 'first, do no harm.'"[1]

I knew Luke needed to get appropriate aftercare.

I explained Luke's history and need for a specialized aftercare protocol. The PA just stared at me like I had two heads. *Does she not understand the severity of this situation?*

"I'll pass along the information to the doctor" was all she said before leaving the room.

"She didn't understand a word you said, Mom," Luke said, disgusted.

"I know," I replied, already calculating my next move.

Time for another email redescribing Luke's condition of high tolerance and his experiences with anesthesia and its ability to trigger a relapse while highlighting the need for possible opioid blockers. Yes, I'd told them before, and yes, it clearly needed repeating. I am not a medical expert but saw the potential disaster looming. To them, I may have been just another meddling mother, but I didn't care.

Mentally prepared, Luke walked into the hospital on October 6, the day of the surgery. Duke's surgical floor was impressive. A large screen informed family members in the waiting room exactly what stage the patient was in: pre-op, transport, surgery, post-op, and post-op consultation. No names—just personal patient codes. Hospital staff armed Jim and me with a beeper alerting us to his status changes during Luke's procedure.

Beep. The staff took Luke back for pre-op.

Beep. I could go into the pre-op area to meet Luke's anesthesiologist. *Great!* I had tons of questions buzzing through my head as I hovered in the small pre-op room awaiting the doctor's arrival. Luke lay calmly in his hospital gown on a bed. I was a nervous mess trying to look brave while my knees buckled underneath me.

The anesthesiologist entered the room, introducing herself. Instead of holding out her hand, she hugged me and said, "I am the chief of anesthesia and the momma of four boys, Mrs. Herrick. I promise to look after your son as if he were my own."

I instantly felt like I could breathe again. "I reviewed the doctor's notes about Luke's high tolerance and his reaction to sedation. I chose this case to ensure all the right drugs will be used. He's in good hands."

"Thank you!" I blurted out. They *had* paid attention!

She then showed me the 25 units of blood packed in an ice chest underneath his bed. She went through the procedural details, ensuring we understood that a tiny nick could cause an instant bleed out, but she assured us they were prepared. My panic returned.

Before leaving, the doctor again reassured me Luke would be fine. She was not just on her game as a doctor but she was also a caring soul. Knowing another mom was in charge comforted me.

The anesthesiologist left the room and gave us a few minutes by ourselves.

"You'll be fine, Bug. This will soon be over," I said, trying my best to reassure him.

"I hope so, Momma. I love you so much."

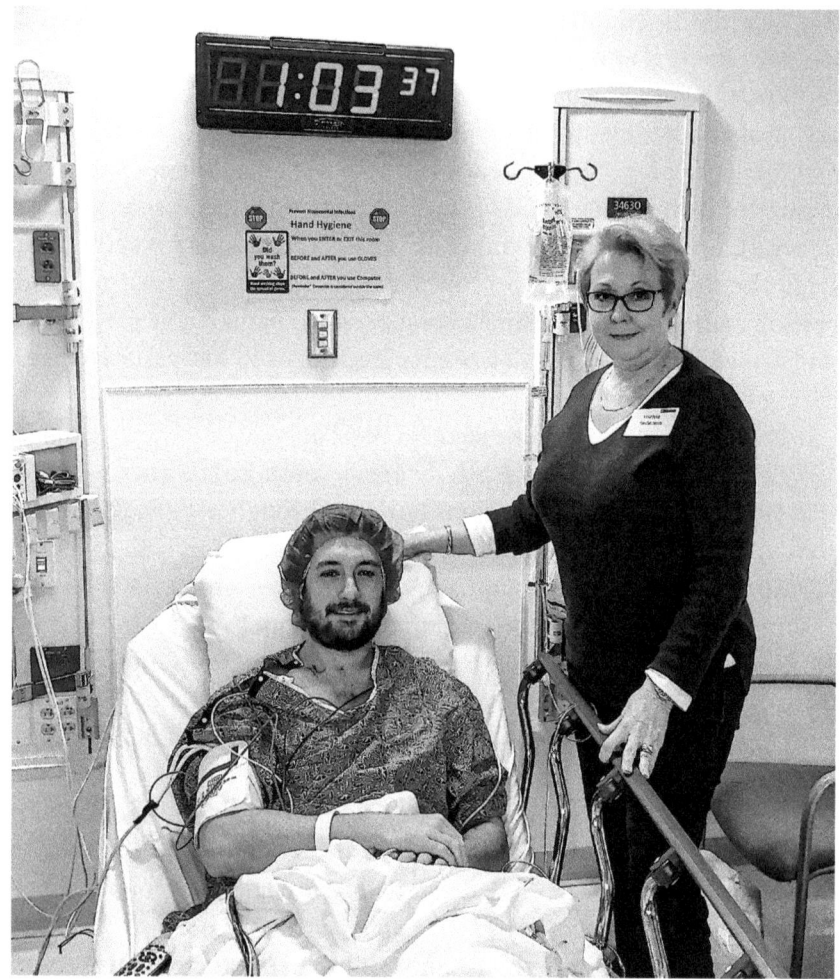

With Luke in pre-op at Duke, 2016. Surgery #4 and counting.

"And I you, child," I replied with a kiss. "More than you know."

I observed my son with great pride. He was brave. After all, this was not his first rodeo, and I had to trust that he was in good hands. I left the room, praying I would see my son again, healthy and whole.

Beep by beep, we followed Luke's progress during the ordeal. The surgery was scheduled for 2 p.m., and we were told it would only take 30 minutes. One hour—no beep. Two hours—no beep. Worry swept over me like a tidal wave. *Perhaps they went right into surgery option number two, and I was not notified as promised. Why is it taking so long?*

Chapter 7. The Unseen Enemy

Being connected to whatever electronic device one chooses is an excellent pacifier and killer of time. My friends Caryl, Jeannette, and Deryle tried to humor me through their texting for most of the day. Leaving them to tend to their own families, I wanted to distract myself by writing.

It's hard to write when you don't feel like it. Sitting in the waiting room of a major hospital waiting for your child's surgery to be over is not conducive to writing. Yet stories are strewn throughout the solemn waiting room, just waiting to be told.

One was an elderly man Jim had made friends with during our wait. His wife was on her 27th kidney surgery. He is pacing. It's easy to imagine him pacing for years as he demonstrates a unique type of peace that is half panic, half zombie. Jim hears the script of the man's story, told many times before, and searches the stranger's face for hope, finding it alive in his eyes. The old man appears glad to have a kind soul to share in his wait. In short order, the man's beeper goes off. The news is not good. A simple procedure to replace a valve needed for survival was thwarted by his wife's heart's decision to beat at a Zulu tribal war pace. Mission aborted. There was a sorrowful look on the man's face when he heard that his wife would probably die soon. Yet he thanked God for the fact he still had her and placed the remaining time in God's hands. The two men hug goodbye as if they are brothers. One can almost see two angels walk him down the corridor to her room, one at his back, the other guiding his feet.

Beep. At 5 p.m., our surgery ended, and I was in full panic mode. Thirty minutes later, the final beeper went off. We were summoned to the consulting cubicle, and Jim went in with me to hear the doctor's report.

Dr. Anderson arrived ten minutes later, looking somber. He began the conversation in a slow, guarded tone. "I'm so sorry, Mrs. Herrick. I tried everything to get it out! It was so embedded.... I truly tried everything...."

I grabbed Jim's arm and blurted out, *"Is he OK?"* dreading to hear he died on the table.

"Oh, yes, he's fine," he replied calmly, "it's just..."

"You need to lead with *that*, doctor!" I gasped, trying to keep from shaking him. "Truly," Jim affirmed.

"Oh, sorry. Yes, Luke is fine and in recovery. As I said, we tried everything to remove the filter, first from the femoral vein and then through the jugular vein. It would not budge. I feared it would tear a hole in the vena cava, so I had to stop."

"Did you go on and do the full surgery?" I asked.

"No. We worked on Luke the entire time. It was too late in the day to assemble the necessary team. We just finished 30 minutes ago."

Disappointed, I asked, "Now what? Do we come back in the morning?"

"We already have Luke scheduled for two weeks from today. And by the way, you were right about his resistance to sedation. He fought it like he was fighting for his life."

He was, I thought to myself. "Thank you, doctor."

Another two weeks? Dang. An hour later, we met Luke in the final recovery room. We told him what had happened. He was devastated.

Luke began to panic to the point of near hysteria. "Mom, they said they would take it out today!" he shouted.

The nurse tried to reassure me. "It must be a reaction to the anesthesia … he'll calm down once it leaves his body."

I've seen this before, I thought. *It was a drug reaction, all right, but not from anesthesia.*

"We'll need enough medication to get him through the next two weeks!" I demanded from the nurse. My nerves were worn thin, and it was showing. Jim tried to calm everyone down.

"Oh, don't worry," she replied, "I have seven days of Percocet for him, along with valium. If his blood pressure stays high, we'll switch to clonidine."

"Seven days of Percocet? That's not enough!" Luke and I said in unison, both of us freaking out. *Why does no one know that treating someone with SUD requires a different pain management protocol after surgery? What was the point of carefully explaining this to the care team beforehand? Had I been speaking into an abyss?*

*****

While Luke waited for his meds to arrive, I snuck outside to call Rebecca to rant about our experience. Her response shocked me.

"Susan, the truth is, a raging drug overdose epidemic is killing over 200 Americans daily and sending thousands to emergency rooms. Most hospitals have avoided offering any form of addiction medicine training for patients who suffer from SUD. Out of the 129,000 medical fellowships offered nationwide, there are hardly any in addictionology. And out of the 5,500 hospitals in the United States, only 18 offer Suboxone.[2] No wonder Luke was overlooked."

"You're kidding me," I responded.

"Listen, Susan," she continued, "reintroducing opioids to a brain in recovery is dangerous on many levels. Even when a person has been sober for an extended period of time, he remains vulnerable to events that trigger a relapse. Studies show that even a brief exposure to a stressor, like surgery, anesthesia, or the introduction to opioids again, could result in an increase in drug-seeking behavior. The cravings and withdrawal make addicts do stupid, dangerous, and illegal things."[3]

"I'm heartsick, Rebecca. Luke's not drug-seeking to get high. He just knows from experience he will need something to keep the uncontrollable cravings from surfacing. His tolerance is so high. He's being given only seven days of Percocet. He's freaked out that it won't be enough. I am too."

"The meds are given according to the pain level of normal patients. Luke had two small incision wounds, which normally require the prescribed dosage he's been given. His back pain may also intensify due to the surgery, which should also be considered. What was totally overlooked was that he has severe SUD."

Tears began to form in the corners of my eyes as I thought back to Luke's struggles. Through sniffles, I said, "Rebecca, he fought so hard for years to win that battle, and now, through no fault of his own, he's forced back into the ring. It's not his fault."

"I know, my friend. I wish I could be of more help. Good luck, and tell me how he fares tonight. I suspect it will be rough," she said solemnly before hanging up.

Luke, Jim, and I left the hospital. Rebecca was right. Luke had a meltdown in our hotel room. A complete, catastrophic, disturbing neurobiological breakdown. I knew his brain was reacting to the Percocet and his PTSD triggered a perceived death threat. Still, I struggled to support him without taking his verbal assaults personally.

Luke focused his pain and his anguish on me. Jim and I watched helplessly as Luke raged. After chiding him for his outbursts, I suggested he call his sponsor. Luke sat at the edge of his hotel bed and made the call. "I don't want to get high, dude! That's what pisses me off. My mom thinks I'm engaging in *drug behavior.*"

I do, honey, I thought. *This is what happens when you get triggered,* I reminded myself.

Suddenly Luke burst into tears, agonizingly telling his sponsor, "I want to go to sleep. I want to not be in pain. I don't want to *feel* this shit! Now I'm going to have to get my stomach cut open again! Why didn't they do that today?"

Luke's tears turned into heavy sobs. As his breath caught short and he continued talking into the phone, my heart tore into tiny pieces. He continued, "They told me they would do it today, and now I have to do it all over again! I'm just here wallowing in pain! I tried to explain it to the pharmacist, but he didn't care!"

I chimed in softly. "Honey, you just have to let the pharmacist tell you what to do."

"Fuck that!" Luke shouted.

"But you've already had the amount he prescribed you."

"Mom! I've only had 10 milligrams! My pain tolerance is used to the amount I was prescribed before. That was more than 100 milligrams a day!"

"But you've been clean for years."

"It doesn't go back down to ground zero, Mother! They won't prescribe me the amount I need because they are afraid I'll get addicted. A little too late for that, don't you think?! I still hurt! That's the problem. That's what sucks!" he shouted.

"Honey, it's setting off your triggers. You knew this would happen."

Luke began sobbing inconsolably into the phone, sputtering broken sentences. He finally shouted, "I just don't want to be in pain, man!"

I turned to Jim, seeking support, and said, "I just can't take it when he's like this. I just can't go through this anymore."

Luke overheard me and shouted, "Fuck you!"

"We'll check in with the doctors tomorrow," I reassured him.

He turned away from me and told his sponsor, "Jesus! My mom is such a bitch! Seriously, dude! Good God! I'm sorry, dude. I'm sorry, man. It's true! She says, 'I'm here for you, I'm here for you.' Then the second I need something, she calls it *drug behavior* and says she can't help! 'I can't have this in my life anymore.' *Drug behavior! Drug behavior!* I'm over here hurting!" Luke's shouts turned again to heavy sobs, tearing at my heart.

I couldn't take it any longer. Finally, I caved. I said, "Honey, just take whatever Percocet you need tonight. I promise we'll see a doctor who can help first thing in the morning."

Jim handed Luke the bottle, and he quickly took one-third of the contents. Within minutes, he calmed down, apologizing to us with remorse, and crashed on the bed, completely exhausted.

*****

I lay awake most of the night, trying to figure out who to contact. An addictionologist would have been the right person to see. Unfortunately, they were pretty much nonexistent. Luke didn't need a psychiatrist. They only treated mental health disorders. Luke was in pain after surgery with insufficient medication. A pain management specialist seemed like the right person to solve Luke's problem.

On our way home early the following day, I called Rebecca back, asking for a favor.

"You were right. Last night was beyond rough. I need an emergency pain management consult for Luke today. Could you refer him?" I asked.

Rebecca happily obliged and made a few calls. Luke and I loaded up in my car, charts in hand, convinced we could find help by going to a local pain management clinic. Luke looked terrible. When we arrived at the pain clinic, he was withdrawn, shaky, and in pain, so I took over the conversation when the nurse came in to make a history file. She never looked at his medical records. After typing in a few notes on her computer, she walked out.

Ten minutes later, an older, humorless doctor came into the room. Again, I went through Luke's surgery and addiction history. He never picked up Luke's medical records.

The man glared at me in a cold, stoic manner, then scoffed, "You're asking me to give your son two weeks of narcotics? Seriously?"

"I am asking for medication management for his craving, sir. My son is chemically dependent. Through no fault of his own, he has been put back on narcotics. He does not react to them like most people."

The doctor just rolled his eyes.

"It is not a choice," I fired back, suspecting he hadn't taken any courses in addiction. With my memory still intact, I spouted, "According to the CDC website, sir, opioids are addictive. In fact, as many as one in four patients receiving long-term opioid therapy in a primary care setting struggles with opioid addiction."[4]

Totally ignoring my comments, he growled, "I'll send him to the methadone clinic."

Seeing that he had yet to open Luke's file, I tried to clarify Luke's situation. "He's going back into surgery in two weeks, doctor; this is not for a walk down. I need someone to manage his pain. The methadone clinic just passes it out. He just had the first surgery yesterday," I softly reminded him, holding back my anger.

"Oh, are you a doctor, ma'am?" he cynically asked, cocking his eyebrow with a smirk.

That did it! Taking offense, I took a deep breath before exploding at his arrogance.

"My advanced degrees are not in a clinical field, but after living with this disease for six years, I have learned a thing or two because *I can read*...."

He glared at me as I pulled out an article from the Anesthesia Patient Safety Foundation by doctors Murphy and Szokol called "Use of Methadone in the Perioperative Period."[5] "These doctors say there have been limited clinical trials of methadone in surgical patients. This is why I am concerned."

At this point, I couldn't tell if he was calculating a learned response or ready to pounce. Hoping I was getting through, I continued.

"From what little literature *I* found, patients can be on methadone on the day of surgery, but it can leave them opioid-tolerant, thus needing additional opioids during and after surgery.[6] This fact concerns me. My son already has a documented high tolerance to opioids, very high." I held up his hospital charts. "Putting him on methadone now may put him at even greater risk for needing more narcotics during and after surgery. I am talking about a major invasive abdominal surgery requiring six weeks of recovery and a pain med walk-down. Plus, he's on a medication that could cause an adverse reaction to methadone. No, I am not a doctor, but it's all in his chart! What is our other option, *doctor*?"

The doctor still never opened Luke's chart. He asked Luke to leave the room so he could talk to me alone. As he walked out, Luke shot me a glance. *Go for it, Momma Bear!*

The doctor glared at me and callously remarked, "Ma'am, your son is a drug addict, and you are his dealer. His brain has been permanently damaged, and it will never recover. He doesn't have a chance. He will *always* be drug-seeking. I suggest you wake up before *you* kill him." With that harsh statement, he opened the door for me to exit the room.

Stunned, dumbfounded, hurt, and enraged, I walked to the car where Luke waited. My body shook with anger—not that the doctor didn't offer help, but that he called Luke a hopeless brain-damaged drug addict. *How can anyone be so callous, so blind to the struggle we've endured?*

Luke reached over to tenderly take my hand and said quietly, "Welcome to my world, Mom."

"Now, what do we do?" I asked, wiping my tears.

"We go back to the streets," he said woefully.

"Oh no, Bug...."

"We're out of options, Mom, and almost out of time. You want to go home and get on your disguise again?" he asked as he pulled out his woolly hat.

"No, Bug, I'm willing to die for you. Prison doesn't scare me. Losing you does. So be it," I replied as I drove to the bank.

Luke made a quick phone call to arrange for a meet-up. To safeguard me, he had a friend come pick him up.

"Be careful, Bug. Please make sure what you are getting is safe," I whispered to him as he walked out of the house.

He turned sadly and said, "I don't want to die, Mom. I just need to survive until the 19th. I will do my best."

Watching him get in his friend's car made me realize not many things scared me anymore, except losing him. Of course, the prospect of him getting busted frightened me, but not for the legal ramifications. Yes, they would be challenging, but knowing he would be put in jail and forced to go through a painful detox without the benefit of any medication in a cold cell without medical support terrified me.

Most jails and prisons around the country forbid Methadone and Suboxone, even when legitimately prescribed, on the grounds that they pose safety and security concerns. Dr. Shabbar Ranapurwala, in *The American Journal of Public Health*, stated, "In the first two weeks after being released from prison, former inmates were 40 times more likely to die of an opioid overdose than someone in the general population."[7]

Even prisons don't withhold insulin from a diabetic.

Luke came back with a small bag tucked inside his shirt. He asked me to keep his pills in our locked safe so he would not be tempted to use more than needed. He then wrote out a dosing schedule for us to follow. Thank God a pharmacist friend dropped off a box of Narcan nasal spray earlier in the year.

I didn't know what Narcan was, so I looked it up on the CDC website. Narcan, better known as naloxone, "is a life-saving medication that can reverse an overdose of opioids—including heroin, fentanyl, and prescription opioid medications—when given in time. Naloxone quickly reverses an overdose by blocking the effects of opioids. It can restore normal breathing within two to three minutes in a person whose breathing has slowed or even stopped due to opioid overdose. More than one dose of naloxone may be required when stronger opioids like fentanyl are involved."[8]

Jim and I took turns at Luke's bedside for the next two weeks, watching him and praying we would not have to use Narcan.

No words could describe what I felt sitting beside my son while he slept. My body buzzed with anxiety; I was terrified that my son could die at any moment. I felt I had to be on guard in full warrior queen mode. I attempted to soothe myself by going to my familiar place of numbness, but my body and mind were in overdrive, trying to find a solution that could help him. I asked myself, over and over, but to no avail, *Why can no one help him? What can I do to support him? Why are there no other options? Why doesn't anyone in the medical community care? Why is this happening?*

Luke seemed so innocent in his sleep. My mind drifted back to those nights I sat beside his crib, hoping to soothe him into a restful sleep. His sharp, sudden jerking, with a pause in his breathing, quickly brought me back to reality. I grabbed the Narcan but then put it back down as he took a deep breath and started snoring. As I sat back in my chair, a quiet prayer escaped my lips. *Please, God, bring my son back. No pain. No drugs. He's been through so much. Let him be free of this terrible disease. Let him be healthy and whole again.*

*****

During the two-week wait, Luke tried hard not to be irritable, but we both knew it was a reaction to the narcotics. Jim organized the paperwork and dealt with the lawyers and insurance company. I lived in my safe place of numb.

Still livid at the treatment we received locally at the pain clinic and the lack of understanding we experienced at Luke's first surgery, I wrote another email to the surgical team, hoping to avert another debacle. There was too much at stake to care if anyone thought me a meddling mother.

Two hours later, I received emails from the team telling me they were assembling a personal surgical protocol and developing a process to care for him postoperatively and outpatient. Luke and I could finally breathe, knowing the appropriate care would be given. Relieved as I was, I was also saddened that I had had to ask for these accommodations. How many other parents lost their child because they didn't know the true nature of their child's disease or even how to ask for specialized care?

On October 18, we checked in at 5:30 a.m., got our beepers, and took our seats in the waiting room. Luke was immediately escorted into pre-op.

Prep was taking a long time because this would be a much more invasive surgery than the first one. We were told to count on four hours. Luke was quite sedated, drifting in and out when my beeper told me I could see him.

The room was full of very serious-looking medical personnel focused on Luke. The new anesthesiologist told me the plan. "Thank you for the email detailing Luke's medical history and challenges. Most chemically dependent people are not so honest, so we cannot treat them as they need. We planned to give him a spinal block to keep his narcotic levels low. Unfortunately, his thoracic fusion restricts us from using a full epidural, but we'll still use a partial block." I nodded, trying to take it all in.

The anesthesiologist's words were comforting. He said, "We are going to do our best. I'm using a different approach utilizing various pain medications to keep morphine to a minimum in his recovery. Ketamine is one. We'll try to keep him on it as long as possible after surgery, but if he starts seeing little green men, let us know, and we'll port over to something else." He winked, asking if I had any more questions. I didn't.

I blew Luke a kiss and told him how much I loved him and would see him in just a few short hours. He gave me a groggy smile and kiss-pucker-smack back in return.

My heart. My love. My Bug. All those tubes, lines, and machines blinking took me back to 2010 and the sheer terror of watching him fight for his life, yet I could feel nothing. Shock. Probably a blessing; if I could feel it, I would have been screaming. Slowly I walked back into the waiting room. For the next four hours, I watched the seconds tick away, one by one, just like I had watched the lines in the highway roll by when Baxter and I drove to Florida after the accident. Honestly, I don't remember much more of that day.

After the last beep, Jim and I made our way to the familiar cubicle and waited for the doctor to give his report.

"Luke's fine!" Dr. Anderson exclaimed, remembering our first post-op exchange. We both smiled in relief. Then he got serious and gave us the details. "Luke did not lose a great deal of blood. The heart and lung machines were not needed. However, I had to cut it out in small pieces—over one hundred."

"One hundred pieces?" I asked, thinking he was exaggerating.

"Yes," he replied. "Over one hundred."

"I'm sorry. Go on, please," I replied, realizing the severity of the surgery.

"He's still in recovery for another two hours, and then he will be transported to his room in the main hospital. A nurse will call you shortly with instructions. I suggest you go to your hotel and relax for a while. You can see him tonight, but I warn you, he's in rough shape."

We thanked him and left to gather our belongings.

Finally, at 6 p.m., we got a call it was OK to go to his hospital room. I was not leaving that night. Ever. Security would have to take me out if need be. Thankfully, I was invited to stay, and staff showed me an oversized chair that turned into a full recliner with a pillow and blanket. It obviously was not their first time dealing with a protective mother.

Luke was still not fully awake when I walked in. Not even close. When he did come to, he'd just grimace in pain. My knees buckled as I peeked at the new 19-inch surgical incision running down his abdomen. It was held together by staples. Medications were pouring into him. Tubes and wires are inserted with precision. Machines were beeping familiar sounds that haunted me from his accident. A thread held my heart together as it was breaking for my son. I felt so hopeless. Mothers always wanted to make it all better, but I had nothing to do.

I set up my makeshift bed beside his and tried to relax. Sleep was not an option. Not tonight. For the next six hours, I stood steadfast as he intermittently reached out his hand, moaning weakly to see if I was still close by.

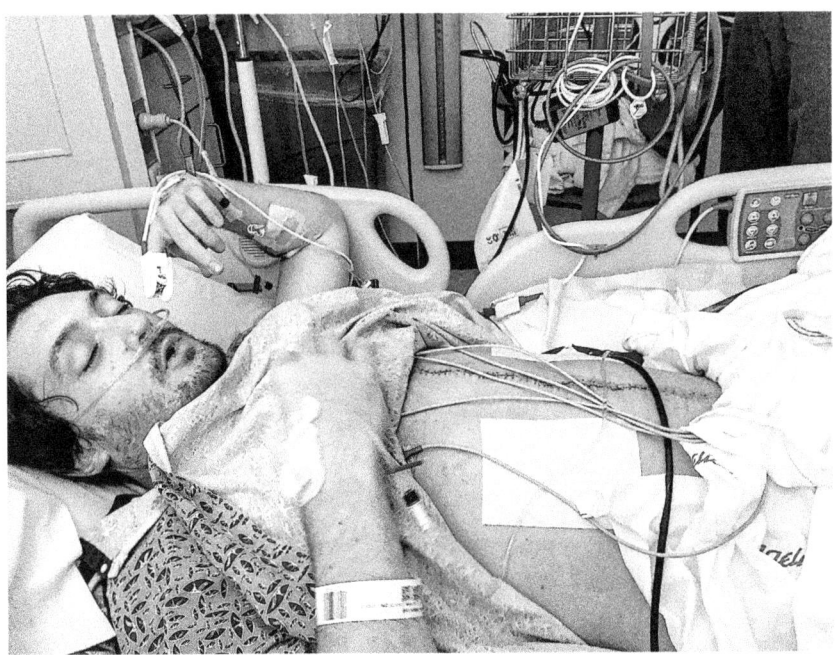

The pain is real. After surgery #4 at Duke.

"I'm right here, Bug. I'm not leaving your side. Just go back to sleep," I would whisper between lullabies.

*****

At 7:00 a.m., the shift changed. At 8:00 a.m., Luke's room filled with new staff reviewing his chart, including a new anesthesiologist who was updated on his specific needs.

"Looks like we have a challenge here," he said thoughtfully, reviewing the paperwork. "We're going to keep Luke on the anesthesia drugs for as long as we can in the hope he will not need a lot of morphine."

"The little green men one?" I asked, forgetting its name.

He laughed. "Mom, I assume?" I nodded. "Yes, Ketamine. It's good at treating acute pain but has dissociative properties that distort perceptions of sight and sound and can produce hallucinations."

"Little green men," Luke moaned. We both smiled, seeing Luke was conscious and alert. Well, almost alert.

The doctor went on with concern, "Luke, I see you've been pushing the morphine drip a lot—more than we hoped for."

"He has a terribly high tolerance and untreated PTSD from a previous accident," I blurted out. *Why could I not keep my mouth shut and let Luke answer for himself?*

"Don't worry, folks. Our main goal is to keep Luke comfortable. He's just been through a very invasive surgery, and I promise we'll do everything possible to keep him comfortable." He turned to Luke before leaving. "Try to use the morphine pump only when you truly need it."

Luke nodded with a groggy smile. "Thank you," he mumbled.

Over the next 10 days, Luke impressed everyone with his immense grit and determination.

On day one, Luke sat in a chair and took a few steps unaided to the bathroom. On day two, he began his daily walks around the corridors. On day three, the Ketamine was stopped as he started seeing little green men and was talking to them.

On day four, Luke's use of morphine kept going up without the Ketamine. Since his blood pressure was very high and he continually spiked a fever without any visible infection, nurses assessed he really was in pain and not drug-seeking to get "the high." His stay was extended from 5 to 10 days.

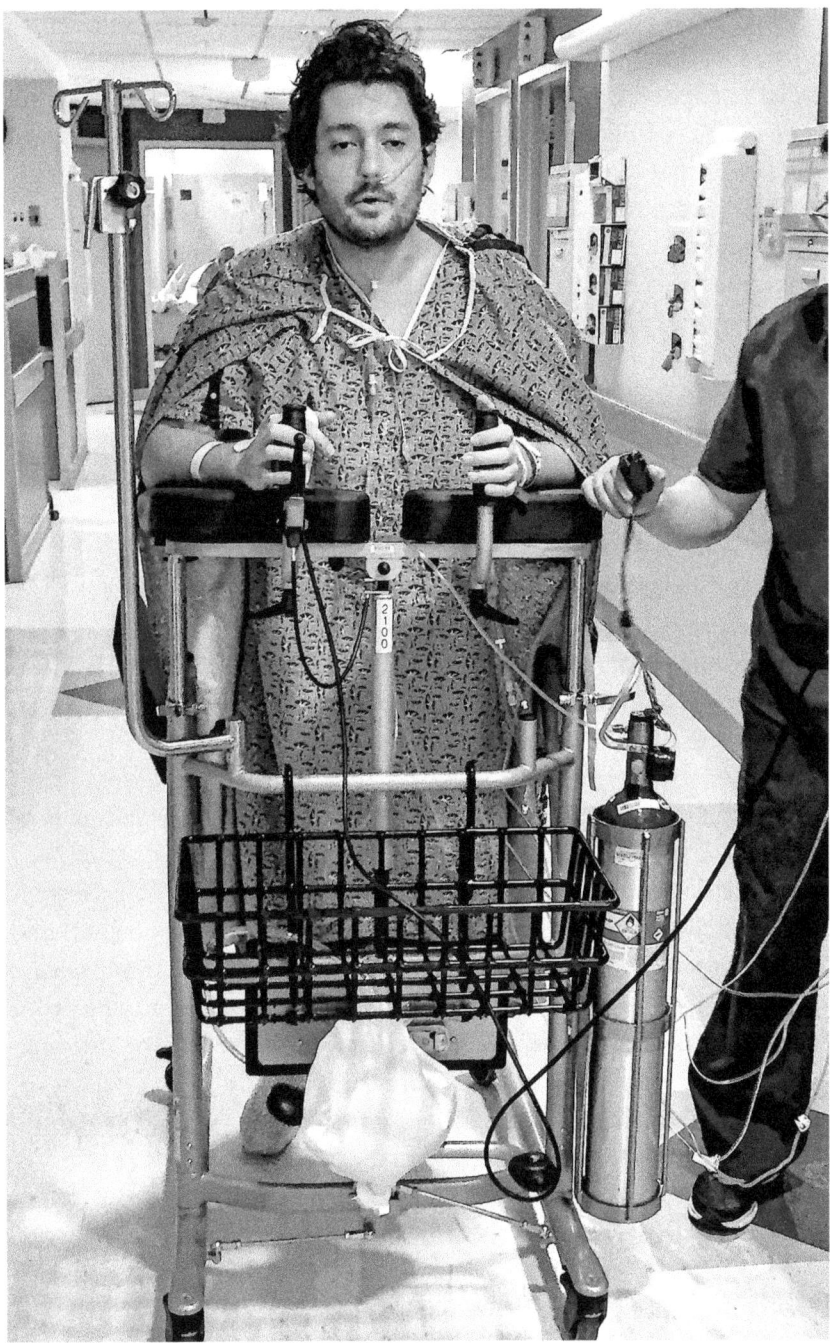

Fighting hard to recover. Luke was singing softly, "I'm dancing in the rain."

Day 8 was enlightening, to say the least. Mid-morning, four distinguished doctors in their scrubs walked into Luke's room. They introduced themselves as the head anesthesiologists in the hospital and came to talk to him regarding his tolerance. I could see by their age and demeanors that the "A team" had been brought in.

The lead doctor introduced the team and then addressed Luke. "Mr. Paschal, we are here to talk to you about the high level of narcotics you are on. The nurses have confirmed you are in intense pain when they try to lower your dosage. We came to personally assess your situation."

The second doctor said, "We have never seen anyone on this high dosage remain conscious. Quite frankly, what you are taking now is enough to put down an elephant, yet here you are, having a coherent conversation with us." They all nodded in concern.

Of course, I felt I had to talk for Luke, even though he was wide awake and capable of speaking on his own behalf. "He has always had a high drug tolerance, including alcohol, as did—"

The doctor cut me off abruptly. "This is beyond high, Ms. Herrick."

Turning to Luke, the head doctor asked, "Luke, we'd like permission to write a paper using your tolerance as a case study."

Luke gave permission. I was busily connecting the dots. They would have quite a challenge getting him down to a safe dosage level for release.

The first doctor continued, confirming my thoughts. "We are gradually switching you to Methadone to get you out of the hospital and to our outpatient pain management clinic. We simply cannot release you using this large dosage of narcotics. The clinic already has your chart and has a team assembled. The nurse will give you the information shortly." They left wishing us both the best.

"Momma?" Luke shot me his pre-panic glance.

I saw Luke's anxiety rising and knew I needed to reassure him.

"Son, we will get you the best help we can, I promise you. You've got great doctors waiting in the wings. Just hang in there. We're a team. You are not in this alone. I promise." *Was I making empty promises again?* Oh Lord, I prayed not.

On day 10, Luke was released with the appropriate medication doses and was happy to be home. Even though he was uncomfortable,

Chapter 7. The Unseen Enemy

he pushed himself daily to be positive. We had his bed ready, but he spent most of his time in a recliner playing Xbox to take his mind off his situation.

*****

A week later Luke had his first post-hospital appointment. Jim and I loaded Luke up in the car and drove to Durham, where the outpatient pain clinic was located. Dr. Bucannon (name changed) was the chief and took over his case personally. This man was our saint.

"Nice to meet you in person, Professor Herrick, Mr. Paschal," he said as Luke and I entered his office.

"Please call me Susan. I'm just the mom here." Luke put on a strong face and shook the doctor's hand, but he was exhausted, gripping a pillow to his midsection.

"I will say you are up on substance use medications, Susan. It is a new field of study. Is Mr. Herrick here? If so, let's invite him in, as I have a protocol involving all the family."

Jim joined us as the doctor brought us notepads and began outlining his plan. "We're going to walk you down on Methadone."

Luke gasped, fearing a harsh withdrawal.

"Don't worry; I have five medications to add to the Methadone making your walk down much less painful. You will not be sent to one of those cold clinics and be made to wait in line. Our goal is to totally walk you off all medications in six weeks. If you have problems or cravings at the end of that time, you will be physically strong enough to go into a treatment center. In the meantime, we will see you weekly for counseling and a medicine check. At least one parent must be with you, as you can't drive while on these meds. Luke, is that OK with you? Jim, Susan?"

We all nodded yes. This man really understood chemical dependency and the need for the entire family to be involved.

Dr. Bucannon then turned to Jim and me and said, "Here is your challenge as parents. All these drugs require different dosages at varying intervals—24/7. Someone must be in charge, and corners cannot be cut. Doing so will cause Luke undue discomfort. I will slowly decrease the dosage each week, meaning you may have to cut some in half or quarters."

Jim agreed to be in charge. The doctor continued, "Please keep all the drugs in a locked safe where you have the key, perhaps always on your person. No offense, Luke, I know you understand."

"My sobriety is very important to me, doctor," Luke replied.

The doctor then took the time to review each medication, stating its purpose and possible side effects. Jim was taking notes, and I could see Luke relaxing, knowing all his concerns had been addressed with concrete solutions about his post-surgical care and psychological and neurobiological problems. For the first time in ages, I felt secure knowing Luke was being treated appropriately.

After we all got settled back in at home, Jim got to work. In a matter of hours, he had all the medications organized in separate distribution containers with the date and time on each bottle. He also created a ledger listing the hour and dosage of all the different drugs so he could administer them and check for compliance. The safe key chain was around his neck and an alarm sat at his side of the bed.

The dosages were lowered weekly as Luke's ill temper intensified.

"Methadone is a dirty drug, Mom," he told me one afternoon as he paced the living room.

"I'm not sure what you mean, Luke." I replied.

"It's a synthetic narcotic with a lid on it. It's still addictive, you know," he snapped back. "I'm on my third enema because I can't poop, I itch all over, I'm sleepy all day and I can't remember anything, plus I feel really nauseous like I want to throw up. I can't even play my Xbox without constantly screwing up."

I didn't know how to reply. I could see Luke was not in the mood to talk. He just needed to express his frustrations.

All in all, Luke was very good at following the protocol, but I could see his anxiety escalating. His moods were changing rapidly, and he was spending more time in his room in the dark which concerned me.

We were all stuck in a state of limbo. The only thing that kept his spirits high was finding out he had one of the filters that would most likely award him a settlement. *But at what cost?* I thought to myself.

By early December, I saw signs of withdrawal from the Methadone despite gradually reducing the doses. Luke was always very tired, restless, and so irritable I could barely talk with him. He also had trouble sleeping and started sweating so much that I washed his sheets daily.

Chapter 7. The Unseen Enemy

On our next trip to Durham, I asked for a private consult with Dr. Bucannon when Luke was in with his counselor. He was more than happy to oblige. I started the conversation with accounts of Luke's behavior and physical reactions to the withdrawal process, sharing my concern that Luke might be unable to successfully walk down on his own.

"I am seeing that also, Susan," Dr. Bucannon replied. "Maybe it's time to start looking for a detox unit and treatment center. I know you are his mother, but Luke is an adult. He must want to go on his own. It's the only way sobriety works."

"I've learned that lesson, sir," I replied, nodding my head. Yet I felt the need to go further and ask his opinion on the bottom line.

"Sir, I would like to ask you for a real, down-to-earth assessment of my son's ability to maintain sobriety from a neurobiological perspective. I mean a long-term assessment. You see, a pain management doctor once told me Luke had permanent brain damage and called him a hopeless drug addict. To me, that means he was pretty sure Luke was doomed to overdose one day. Was he right? Were those just words I didn't want to hear because Luke is my son?" I asked, trying to hold back the tears.

Dr. Bucannon grimaced. "I am so sorry. There is no excuse for a doctor ever telling anyone those words. There is no such thing as a hopeless drug addict, Susan. It's a disease just like cancer or diabetes. Those illnesses have different types and stages, just like substance abuse. Just like with cancer, there are many variables and outcomes."

I nodded with hope, reminding him, "Luke's is severe because of the accident and now this surgery."

Dr. Bucannon acknowledged my statement but went on cautiously to explain, "It doesn't matter if one gets addicted due to experimentation, or an injury, or by accident. The end result is that the brain reacts to the drugs in the same way. It's not the person's fault. It's a neurobiological response that does not single out the good guys from the bad guys. Addiction does not make judgments—people do."

"Isn't that the truth," I replied in agreement, feeling again the judgment from the lunch ladies.

Dr. Bucannon went on. "Your son's addiction is severe, but many get sober and stay that way, living long and productive lives. It takes commitment, a community of support, a healthy lifestyle, and maybe MOUD."

"What is MOUD?" I asked, hearing this term for the first time.

"Medications for opioid use disorder."

"Like Suboxone?" I asked, connecting the dots.

"Yes. Methadone, Buprenorphine, which is Suboxone, or Naltrexone. Many adults have overcome a substance use problem with or without these drugs. That is a testament to the fact that not only is addiction recovery possible, but it's also common. That's not to say there may not be relapses, which happen more often than not. But if the desire remains without too many stressors, they can make it."

"OK, but I also read that it's a lot harder to maintain sobriety when there are additional conditions like the ones Luke has: severe anxiety, a high tolerance, genetics, and PTSD. Plus, Luke recently lost his father and lives in chronic pain due to his spinal fusion. Now we have the trauma and added drugs from this surgery."

I paused before asking the next question ... I knew I was starting to ramble. Taking a deep breath, I went on to address my greatest fear. "I guess what I am asking is, are his chances at maintaining sobriety long-term the same as the ones you just talked about? I mean, like those people without all these other conditions, mental health disorders, and genetic predispositions?"

Dr. Bucannon dropped his head before answering. I could tell he was choosing his words cautiously. "Susan, your son is high-risk and dual diagnosis, but it is possible."

"I want the hard-core truth, sir, as if you were asking about your son. I need to know how to proceed in my life and how to help Luke the best I can without enabling him. Luke is my heart, my everything, and I need to know ... is he terminal?" The tears started to flow. Dr. Bucannon reached out for a tissue for me.

"Susan," he started, "I'll be honest with you. We both know no one has a crystal ball. SUD is a chronic illness, meaning it has no cure, but we can treat it. We don't use the term terminal, but since you asked ... Luke is high-risk, and I won't lie to you: his midbrain has been severely compromised due to the sheer number of narcotics he has been on. And yes, his triggers like stress, PTSD, and anxiety make it more challenging. He would benefit from anxiety medication as anxiety is a huge trigger for Luke, but he was addicted to many of them when he was younger, complicating the matter. The brain does not forget. The fact is Luke's brain no longer functions normally without the drugs, and this imbalance can take time to heal. Much of the damage can be reversed with prolonged abstinence. I won't lie to you; some of the damage in the midbrain could be life-long. His receptors may not heal entirely, but that does not mean he is doomed. Do you hear me?" he said with deep sincerity, reaching across the table to take my hand.

I nodded, wiping away the tears, then asked, "So … where do we go from here?"

"Luke needs to detox, go to treatment, and stay in an environment that supports his sobriety. No more drugs, surgeries or trauma. He needs a clean diet, meditation, exercise, nutritional support, and a calm lifestyle."

I laughed. "Oh, good luck with that one—Luke's been jumping off cliffs since he was a kid. Drama is his middle name—just like his momma, I'm afraid." We both smiled.

Dr. Bucannon finished up by saying, "Luke truly wants his sobriety. I am convinced of that fact. Unfortunately, his brain chemistry and neurological responses are not in his favor, but that does not mean he does not have a chance at a wonderfully productive life. *Never give up hope on that young man!* He's smart. He has dreams and goals. He will have to give it his all, and you've got to know the longer he has sobriety, the more his brain can heal. How much is not in our control. Your job is to encourage and support his efforts without enabling him. OK?"

"OK," I whimpered as he gave me a long hug and more Kleenex.

Thankfully Luke slept most of the way home, so he didn't see the tears streaming down my face. I grieved the times I blamed him for not controlling his anxiety, thinking it was just a matter of willpower, not knowing a part of his brain was circuited to run hot. I hated myself for thinking he was just an uncaring teen, not understanding all those raging hormones, prescribed drugs, and heartbreaks were contributing to his behavior. I was so embarrassed for raging at him after his first sobriety, for not trying hard enough when I did not heed the warning of the professionals that he needed more time for his brain to heal.

I suppose I had always thought deep in my heart that once Luke stopped using the drugs, his brain would return to normal, and so would our lives. Poof. Healed. I thought it was just a matter of willpower and working the 12 steps. That may be true for some, but maybe not for my son. Now I knew the facts from an expert, and I could proceed with the truth, as painful as it was to hear. On that trip home, I vowed to give Luke whatever care and support he needed without enabling him and make as many beautiful memories as possible, just in case. Even if the odds were not in his favor, I accepted that he could beat them and vowed never to cave into fear.

*****

First things first, however. I had to convince Luke it was time to go to yet another rehab. In his right mind, that would be easy. He knew the score. This was not his first dance with the devil. Luke's brain, however, was now addicted to Methadone, and he was falling into drug addict mode. He once told me being under the influence was like driving a bus with a monkey on his back, one of its hands covering his eyes and the other trying to grab the wheel.

It was now time to get that monkey off his back. However, getting him to agree to treatment would be easier said than done. That monkey was not about to leave on its own.

Luke fought the idea of going back into rehab. The drugs again hijacked his brain and drug-seeking behavior was starting to emerge. This was not a conscious decision. He wasn't thinking about getting high; he was simply seeking relief from the cravings and pain of withdrawal, and this was how his brain processed that need. Anger, bargaining, denial, and depression cycled daily.

Putting anyone in a treatment center needs its own set of instructions posted on every recovery website. Most people do not know how to proceed when a family member or loved one needs help. You usually just don't show up at the door of the treatment center, especially if the person afflicted does not want to go. It takes planning and an intervention team.[9]

The purpose of an intervention is to confront the person and show him how his drug use is hurting him, as well as his friends and family, and then to get him to admit that he needs help. It is usually directed by a credentialed alcohol and drug counselor, but we didn't have one available, and the treatment center was two hours away. Since I knew the

Chapter 7. The Unseen Enemy

ropes after our previous encounters, I put my strong team together and went into action.

Our first step was to call a local treatment center to ensure it had a bed for Luke and that insurance would cover his stay. The insurance approved our request within the hour, and the co-pay was settled. In short order, all the paperwork was in place—minus Luke and his signature.

Without Luke's knowledge, Jim and I called Worth and a dear friend, Deryle, to come to the house to confront Luke. I hoped to convince him the only way back to his successful life before the surgery was to go to rehab. Since Luke had been unwilling to go when I spoke with him earlier, I knew an intervention was the only way to get through to him. We set a date: 7:00 p.m., December 13.

I'm not going to lie; it was not a pretty scene. Luke felt attacked, ganged up on, and humiliated, putting him on the defensive. His first reaction was explosive, and he threatened to leave. Luke would have shoved past me and left the house if it had been just me. That's why a team is needed, not just a close family member. Deryle sat close to him to calm his anger. He loved her and was held in check by that fact. One by one, we gently told Luke how much we loved him, cared about his well-being, and how his actions hurt him and all of us, kindly but firmly reinforcing that nothing good could come from his refusing treatment.

It took an hour, but Luke finally broke down, knowing what we said was right. He wanted help and acknowledged a medical detox with in-house treatment was the only way to get it. He was just so afraid of the detox pain again. I was crying as we went into his room to pack his bag. Meanwhile, Jim had the car waiting in the driveway. Everyone hugged Luke goodbye, promising to see him in January when he got out.

On the way to the treatment center, Luke texted his AA brothers in LA, telling them where he was going. Support came from all his friends that night. Support without judgment gave Luke the added determination he needed to move forward. I watched him regain his composure from the rearview mirror. By the time we arrived, he had regained hope and was ready to take on the demon again.

We reached the treatment center, where an intake team was

waiting, a little after midnight. They gave us a few minutes to say our goodbyes. Luke, the man—not the frightened boy—took me by the shoulders, consoling me as my tears flowed with exhaustion and grief.

"I'm going to beat this, Mom. I'll get up with you in a few weeks, and you'll be proud of me again, I promise," he said in full warrior mode.

"I am always proud of you, Luke," I replied. "Not having the guts to come here would be the failure. You are one of the strongest men I know! Nothing will change my love and support for you. Ever! You are my Bug."

"Thank you, Momma Bear. Always and forever," he said, pulling me close.

"Always and forever, Bug," I replied with a kiss, letting him go.

As hard as it was watching Luke walk into the center's dark doorway, I knew it was our only hope. I say "our" because addiction is a family disease. If Luke went down, so would I.

Jim and I drove back home in silence, letting Christmas carols on the radio calm the night. Christmas was always a magical time for me, but now it held only heartache and fear. I was living the true advent—waiting in the darkness for the light to appear and save us.

I could not bring myself to attend church on Christmas Eve without Luke. It was just too painful. All I would see were the ghosts of Christmases past in the darkness. Jim and I stayed home, watched old movies, and went to bed early. My present was knowing we could drive down to see Luke for a few hours on Christmas Day and bring him one gift.

Thankfully the treatment center was just two hours away. We checked in Christmas morning and signed a contract not to interfere with its rules. Before we could see Luke, we had to sit through a one-hour lecture by a nurse telling everyone there how to help our loved ones maintain their sobriety. Vigorous exercise was heavily encouraged, as was clean eating, ensuring the brain got the best nutrition. Much to my surprise, she told us that those who go back to diets heavy on sugar can relapse within weeks; for some addictions, like alcohol, it lights up the brain, causing cravings.[10] *Well, who knew?*

The moment came, and we met Luke in the cafeteria, our present to him in hand. Much to my delight, Luke gave us a great gift. There he was, standing strong, clean, and energized. My son was back.

"I'm killing it, Mom!" Luke exclaimed.

During the afternoon, we learned from the staff that Luke had taken over a leadership position in his groups, and they all bragged about his ability to help others see the need for working the program. Luke beamed with pride. He had also made friends with many of the men there, along with Sandy, a beautiful young nurse. A petite blonde, of course.

Before we left, we watched him shoot a few hoops. I could see that his body had healed physically, and he was ecstatic that with the filter gone his lower back no longer hurt. We were told he would be released a few days after the new year and could come home or stay in a sobriety house in Wilmington.

Leaving that evening, I felt good knowing Luke was back on his game. Now, on to a new year—one good new year, hopefully without mishap and calamity.

Chapter 8

Broken Policies

"A proud man is always looking down on things and people; and, of course, as long as you are looking down, you cannot see something that is above you."—C.S. Lewis

During the last week of treatment, Luke decided to live in a sobriety house in Wilmington as he was now connected to the NA community there. I felt very comfortable with his decision as I knew sober friends would benefit him. One good way to keep sobriety is to have new playgrounds, new playmates, and new toys. This sounds like a simple phrase, but science backs it up as returning to familiar situations can trigger a relapse.[1]

Jim and I drove down for the graduation ceremony the following week. That afternoon the three of us celebrated by going out to lunch. We then drove around to check out the sobriety houses with rooms available. There were three houses from which to choose. We were disappointed that all were in run-down areas; one neighborhood looked dangerous. These homes differed from those in California, which were nestled in safe, lovely residential areas.

There is so much prejudice regarding those in recovery. "I don't want any druggie living next to me" is the sentiment. Don't get me wrong, no one wants to live close to someone with the potential to harm or rob you, and granted, many men in these houses may have done harmful things to others when they were actively using. But that is not who they are now. Yet the prejudice remains because people are uneducated or unwilling to open their hearts.

The fact is sobriety houses demand drug tests of every resident. They also require the occupants to attend regular meetings where the 12 Steps are emphasized and encouragement is given. Some houses even sponsor AA/NA meetings and use MOUD. The participants are good people who fell into the trap of addiction but have taken steps to reclaim their purpose and move toward a healthy and productive future.² A drug and alcohol counselor with

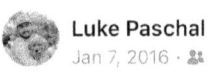

Luke Paschal
Jan 7, 2016

I'm a riser
I'm a get up off the ground, don't run and hider
Pushing comes a-shovin'
Hey I'm a fighter
When darkness comes to town, I'm a lighter
A get out aliver, out of the fire
Survivor

Luke never gives up.

36 years of sobriety once told me that one would be hard-pressed to find a more spiritual person than someone in recovery. Her favorite saying was, "Religion is for those who are afraid of hell. Spirituality is for those who have been there."

By the end of the day, Luke made his choice and moved in. After a nice dinner at the ocean, Jim and I drove back to Southern Pines. I knew Luke could handle himself, and I could see he needed to be on his own again without Momma. It was a new chapter for him, one filled with possibilities.

Luke was also looking forward to driving up to the mountains with Sandy at the end of the month to go to the regional AA convention. It would be three days of speakers, sober parties, and fellowship. When Luke was living in LA, he told me about some of the great parties the AA/NA community threw all over town. They had the same fun and excitement as a regular nightclub—just without alcohol or drugs. There were even glitzy sobriety tents at the Oscars and other glam Hollywood events, as many celebrities are in recovery yet want to party without distraction.

Later in the week, Sandy drove Luke to Southern Pines so we could meet her and so they could pick up Luke's car. I liked Sandy. She was educated, intelligent, and very sharp-witted. No wonder Luke and she connected—she kept him on his toes. Moreover, she had been sober for more than five years. Luke's sober friends always gave me a feeling of security. I gave him his car keys with our blessing.

With Luke settled, Jim and I decided to attend the annual Shaklee meeting near San Francisco. We needed a break too. On the long flight from Raleigh to San Francisco, my mind wandered through the heartbreaking stories of people I knew who personally lived with SUD.

Wanda and I met sailing. We swapped "son stories" with pride and concern while soaking up the rays. Suddenly her demeanor changed as she spotted Luke out on the paddleboard. She leaned back and quietly told me why her son Jon was not on the trip with us.

Like Luke, Jon was a delightful young man with a bio-neurological history, ADD, anxiety, a family history of addiction, and high energy. Jon's high school talent was football. He was injured early on and introduced to Oxycontin. The drug fog added to the fact that he had a documented learning disability, dyslexia, that kept him from maintaining the GPA needed to stay on the team. Because of that, Jon was dropped from the team, leaving him feeling worthless, ashamed, and filled with self-loathing. He started using drugs to self-medicate. After the usual denial and trauma of dealing with teenage addiction, he went into recovery with his parents' complete love and support.

Jon maintained his sobriety for years after treatment, found the love of his life, and took on a calling as a youth counselor in a large, active church. When the church elders found out he and his fiancée were expecting a baby before the ceremony, they kicked him out in disgrace. Many young men in heartbreaking situations go to a bar and drown their sorrows. Jon's brain, however, instantly craved the only substance he had ever known to ease his pain. Just one relapse is all it took to end his life and forever decimate the hearts of those he left behind.

Wanda's story reminded me of a neighbor whose son overdosed. I was walking the dogs early one morning when I heard muffled, anguished screams from down the street. Three minutes later, police cars careened into the neighborhood. Ten minutes later, an emergency vehicle arrived without blazing lights. Jim later found out that the 24-year-old son of a prominent minister was found dead by his mother. All was hush-hush—no one was allowed to reveal the cause. Two days later, gossip was that the boy was laid out in a tiny church in the country. I was ill with the flu, so Jim went by himself to offer our condolences. No one was there. Just an open casket in a darkened sanctuary. Jim sat with the lad for an hour to pay his respects, hoping someone would come. No one did. No signatures in the book except Jim's. The young man was laid to rest the next day without a formal service.

Chapter 8. Broken Policies

Luke's friend Sandy had become addicted to narcotics in nursing school. She hid it for years and could function well in nursing, much like the character Dr. Gregory House on the TV show *House*. Her world came crashing down one morning when she found her best friend had overdosed in their apartment. Sandy was so shaken she voluntarily went into treatment and told her parents. They instantly disinherited her as they were terrified her drug abuse would cause her father to lose his high-powered law clients in New York and pollute her younger brother, who adored her. Banned from her family, she set out on her own in North Carolina for treatment and then worked as a nurse in rehabs and treatment centers contingent upon passing drug tests.

My heart had gone out to her as I could see she loved being accepted into our home and family without prejudice. There was a sadness about her, though. I could only imagine her heartbreak at being cast out of her family for wanting treatment while at the same time watching her father constantly cheat on her mother without consequence. Sandy was the one who chose recovery yet was punished for it.

Unfortunately, six weeks after she and Luke broke up, she hooked up with an old boyfriend who was using. Before long, she was back on drugs, which numbed her heartache. Tragically Sandy overdosed that summer. No obituary, her Facebook profile wiped clean. Her parents erased any footprint of her life.

Why do we believe sins are ranked, filed, and color-coded? How can a parent's ego override their love for their child? When will our love be stronger than our belief system?

*****

Getting away was good for both Jim and me. We spent three days with our friends and colleagues at the convention and ended our trip sightseeing in the city. Walking past one of the piers one morning, I reminisced about Luke's last birthday when we celebrated with Jacob. Little did I know that at that very moment, Luke was being rushed to the hospital with an intestinal blockage.

The doctors warned us a blockage might happen after Luke's surgery. The scarring from the 19-inch abdominal incision could affix itself to Luke's intestine, causing it to crimp and back up into the stomach, which is precisely what happened. Luke woke up writhing in pain, vomiting green fluids, and crying out for help. The men in the house called 911.

Treatment for an intestinal blockage is narcotics for pain and fluids for hydration, both intravenously, as one can't swallow or eat anything without throwing it back up immediately. Then an NG tube (nasogastric tube), a long, flexible plastic tube, is inserted into the person's nose and threaded into the stomach to suck out the contents to relieve the excruciating pain of the blockage. Quite nasty, to be sure.

I panicked after a housemate called two days after the event and grabbed the next flight out. By the time I arrived Luke was ready to be released from the hospital. He had gone four days without food or water and was exhausted. More than that, the morphine instantly triggered cravings. Much to my dismay, he was offered no step-down medications, so he went to a kratom tea shop. He was told by a housemate that kratom worked as well as Suboxone or Methadone without all the nasty side effects. I had never heard of it before.

I was furious but knew nothing could be done to change the facts: one cannot go through an intestinal blockage without a pain killer—it would be inhumane. *But now what? Damn it!*

I immediately called the insurance company for clearance to get Luke back into detox at the treatment center. I was unsure of this kratom tea thing, but I knew if he was back under the care of a team of doctors, they could walk him off, allowing him to get back on his feet, hopefully without cravings. Imagine my shock to find out that Tricare insurance only allowed one treatment stay per 12 months.

"You've got to be kidding me!" I railed at the unfortunate representative on the other end. "My son was not out getting high; he was in recovery after a gruesome, necessary surgery, and then he had another medical emergency, an intestinal blockage, which called for narcotics. It was not his choice. He needs help to walk off the morphine."

"Ma'am, I am sorry, I can't do anything about it. That is the policy—only one treatment center or detox per 12 months." Click.

Can you imagine having chemo for cancer, going into remission only to have it resurface four months later and being told, "I'm sorry, we treated you once already this year. You are on your own for another eight months"? Or having two heart attacks in one year and the emergency room saying, "We saved you once this year; too bad this time around."

Chapter 8. Broken Policies

Why does this happen? Stigma, ignorance, and public policies are based on the unscientific and inhumane view that substance use disorder is a moral failing, not a disease.

Again, here we were in 2016 with an uninformed hospital staff not medically qualified to give Luke Methadone during or after his blockage and Suboxone afterward. Opioids they can prescribe, but Suboxone needed an X-waiver, and no one on staff had bothered to get it. *It's only an eight-hour course,* I screamed inside. Without insurance for medical intervention, we had few options. Luke's only option was kratom tea to ward off the cravings.[3]

Luke would not be allowed to stay in the sobriety house while taking his tea because it has mild opioid properties. Like Suboxone, the tea kept him from craving drugs, but that was a moot point. With great disappointment, we packed his bags and drove him back home, taking him away from new friends and an established support system.

Within five days, Luke was back in the hospital with another blockage.

We arrived in the ER late evening, with Luke grimacing in pain. The nurse on staff was very skeptical of Luke's condition. I could tell he thought Luke was just another addict seeking drugs and was quite harsh with him. I knew from experience that most doctors in the ED think people with SUD are just junkies.[4] Truthfully, I had the same suspicions and thought maybe the tea was losing its ability to cut his cravings. But after looking at his fresh scar, Luke was scent for a CT scan.

After three hours the nurse came back with a kinder demeanor. "Mr. Paschal, indeed you do have a 30 percent blockage." He shot Luke up with morphine on the spot, telling him, "We're going to admit you and put in an NG tube." Luke gladly accepted the pain relief while I put my head back on the chair, trying not to cry.

Again, a blockage was considered a treatable ailment. But if Luke had come in for his cravings, he would have been admonished and sent home with Advil and maybe a referral to the substance abuse clinic the next day for group therapy. In other words, the hospital would not treat his SUD as a disease. I wondered how many other illnesses it deemed unworthy of the Hippocratic Oath.

Luke was admitted in a state of disbelief that this was happening again. He was in the hospital for seven days this time, without water or

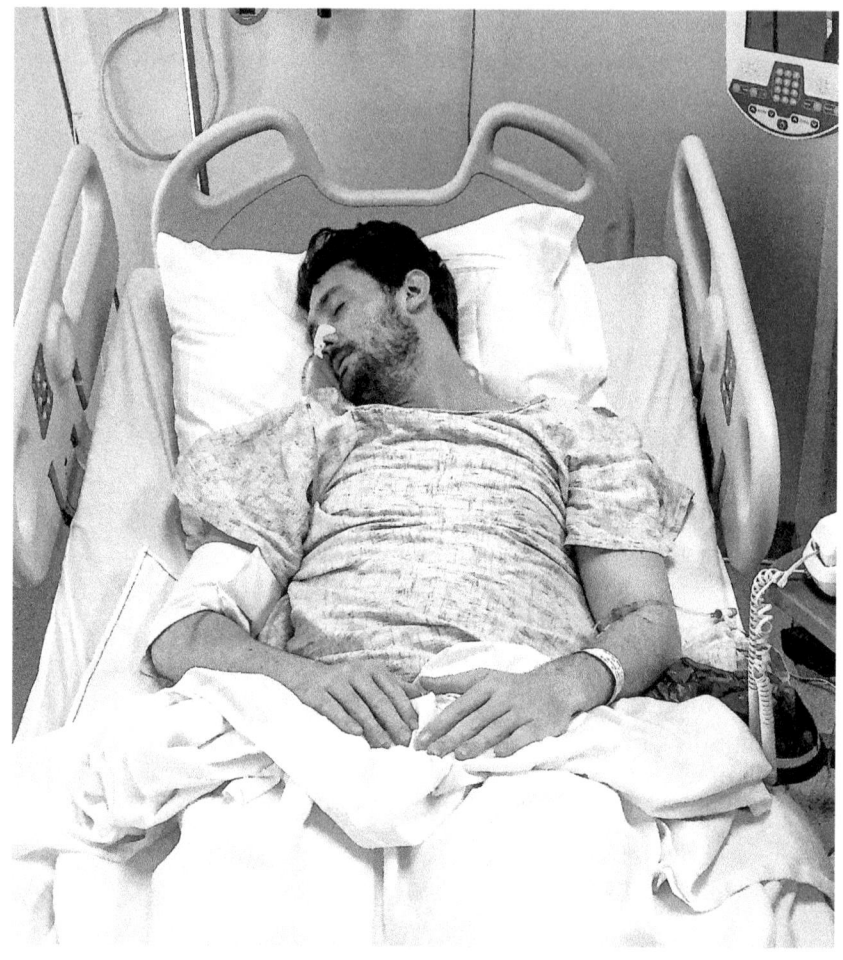

Luke's first blockage with NG tube and morphine onboard.

food, waiting for the blockage to clear. If the NG tube didn't work, he would need another surgery as an intestinal obstruction can cut off the blood supply to part of your intestine, causing the intestinal wall to die. Tissue death can cause a tear in the intestinal wall, which can lead to infection, which can lead to death.

While waiting and praying for all of Luke's body parts to fix themselves, I watched his morphine levels rise due to his tolerance. He was visibly in pain. Every day the staff capped his dosage and fussed at him for saying he was still in pain. I asked that he be ported over to Methadone like had happened at Duke, but no one showed up for a consult.

Chapter 8. Broken Policies

Getting to the end of my rope, I had to storm over to the behavioral care clinic and demand someone come and help. *Enough was enough!*

Luke fought the idea of going back on Methadone. He had experienced harsh side effects before and could not walk down on his own. I begged him to give it another try until his blockage pain was over. To sweeten the pot, I enticed him with a trip to Cabo. Jim and I were scheduled for a business trip there in April.

My request for the Methadone tablets he had been given before was denied, forcing us to be at the clinic at eight o'clock every morning for a shot of the liquid form of Methadone. Luke asked that I go with him the first time as he felt weak after losing another 15 pounds.

The Methadone clinic was not as lovely as the rest of the hospital campus. The little building was pushed back into a wooded area. The parking lot was packed when we arrived, with a line wrapped partway around it. The large waiting room was painted a hideous green and looked as dispassionate as the staff. It was a far cry from the hospital's main lobby, which had coffee, cookies, and smiling volunteers making sure everyone was happy. Inside sat scores of people in sad shape. Many patients were shaking, unshaven, poorly dressed, looking depressed and discarded. One by one, names were called to the front station, where the patients signed in and were given a single dose of the nasty-tasting medication in a paper cup. The nurse made sure they emptied the cup before they were dismissed.

Luke's only words after his dosage were, "This is no way to live, Mom. I feel like a discarded addict." I had to admit I agreed with him, but it was all that was offered.

After one week of the drill, Luke came home and announced he was done with the clinic and was porting back over to kratom tea. The side effects of the Methadone were again harsh, and he experienced nausea, vomiting, constipation, headaches, confusion, mood changes, and terrible itching. It was his decision as an adult, so I didn't try to talk him out of it. Instead, I did a little research to learn more about this kratom tea.

I went to the online, to Kratomtea.com, and read: "Kratom is a tropical plant related to coffee trees grown mainly in Southeast Asia. It contains a chemical called mitragynine, an alkaloid that acts on the brain's opiate receptors and alters mood. In Asia, where use has long been widespread, people use it in small doses as an energy and mood booster, similar to coffee use in the West. They use larger amounts for pain or recreationally, like beer and wine."

It was natural. Good. I liked that. What was disappointing, however, was to read that there had been little research on the tea. Without research, it's challenging to know the full risks.

Back to my Internet search. I was encouraged when I read the opinion of Chris McCurdy, Ph.D., a professor of medicinal chemistry at the UF College of Pharmacy, based on a recent study. "There have been a lot of anecdotal reports suggesting kratom has some pain-relieving properties and has helped transition users from prescription opioids to this product. Scientifically, this becomes one of the most important kratom studies released showing support as a potential treatment option for opioid withdrawal syndrome or opioid use disorder."[5]

Other doctors were firmly against it, stating since there was no lid on it like Suboxone, it could lead to a relapse. My guess was Luke could fall in that second category, but for now, it seemed like the best alternative.

Luke and I sat down for a chat. "Son, I don't know what to say. You look calm and relaxed and say it curbs your cravings. But I'm afraid with your tolerance, it may cause you problems."

"I don't seem to have any other options right now, Mom. My goal is to wean down just like I would on Methadone," Luke stated simply. "Besides, it's giving me the freedom to go to Cabo with you. Let's just go and have a good time and please stop worrying about me," he said, reaching out to give me a hug.

Right. Like I could stop worrying if I wanted to, I thought to myself as we started packing.

Our business went well that year, so we attended the Shaklee training conference in Cabo San Lucas. Luke was very excited to go with us as he knew a few younger people in the group. I was excited for him too. He had been battered and bruised for almost a year without being around friends and enjoying activities. He deserved some fun in the sun, as did we.

*****

Chapter 8. Broken Policies

Had I been thinking things through, I would have remembered that Mexico has pharmacies open to the public with no need for a medical script. And then there was the temptation to join friends his age who liked to drink and party. The trip turned into a bad situation quickly.

Luke returned to the hotel the second night with dilated pupils—a sign of barbiturate use. I could tell he also had been drinking. His personality changed. I could see he had had enough of Mom telling him what to do and just wanted to live a little. I was panicked, knowing the combination could cause an overdose. When his friends came to the room, I railed at them for enabling him. Clueless, they claimed they would just keep an eye on him and went out the door.

Luke kept out of sight for most of the trip. He'd stay out all night partying and sleep on the beach in a far-off cabana most of the day. I was terrified of him overdosing. Granted, he was not on opioids, but the mixture of alcohol and Xanax could be just as lethal. Heaven only knows what else he may have been taking. Yet I was helpless, watching the train speed toward the cliff, praying he would survive the crash.

At sunrise, I scoured the beach looking for him, as he never returned to the room. When I found him, he was exhausted but conscious, telling me he was fine. Arguing was useless. He was alive, and for that moment, that was all that mattered.

Relieved yet destroyed, I crashed into despair and headed to my room for a good cry. On the way there, my business colleagues Moyra and Pam crossed my path covered in sunscreen and wearing smiles. They took one look at me, grabbed my arms, and dragged me along with them to the pool.

"You need help, girl," Moyra stated with love and authority. "You've got to get off this roller coaster or it will take you down too. Trust me, I know."

"I'm trying," I replied, trying to keep myself together. "You don't know what it's like," I mumbled.

"Yup, I do. Same monkey, different circus," she said flatly as we made our way to the pool chairs.

Pam chimed in, "Susan, I almost lost my kid to a mental health disorder. You are not alone. Let us help you."

We spent the day in the pool talking, crying, sharing stories, praying, and laughing off the stress. They were such godsends and helped me remember that even though I loved Luke, it was his addiction, not mine. He alone was responsible. Even though he had been through hell and back, his addiction didn't care, and he would have to take charge of his recovery. My God, it was nice not to be judged for once.

At the end of the trip, I was amazed at how many people came to me with compassion and support, telling me their family stories of addiction. Luke may have gotten back on drugs during the trip, but I had found a renewed strength to continue my life and reset the boundaries. I felt like such a failure, living in shame and constant terror. In short, I saw many parents suffer in silence as the stigma of addiction was too great for many to seek help themselves.

The trip home was somber. Luke was a mess, filled with remorse and self-loathing. Jim was quiet, not knowing how to respond. I was resolved to help Luke find a cheap detox and get him back into a long-term sobriety house. It was clear to me that this route would be his only hope.

No intervention was needed this time. Luke took full responsibility for his actions. He had cravings, and instead of calling a sponsor, he caved. Luke needed a break from hospitals, procedures, and pain, and he wanted to have a good time like everyone else. But he wasn't like everyone else, and he knew it.

Checking the internet, I got a tip about a free detox center in a neighboring county. No reservations; one just showed up hoping a bed would be vacant. Some people lived in their cars in the parking lot, waiting for a spot. It was worth a try, so the day after we got home, Luke and I packed a bag and took off early in the morning to wait in line. Luckily a bed opened that afternoon, and I once again drove away, leaving him to detox.

One week later, I went back to get him.

"So how was detox this time?" I asked as he climbed into the car.

"Just peachy, Mom. They gave me Phenobarbital to calm my anxiety and Seroquel to help me sleep. While I shook and sweated it out, we watched movies, and they checked in to see I was still alive every few hours. Same old, same old."

"We need to talk, Bug. You almost killed yourself, you know…"

Chapter 8. Broken Policies

"You think?" he fired back at me.

Just as I was about to launch into my motherly lecture, he exploded. Not in anger, mind you, but in sheer frustration and grief.

"Don't you think I know that, Mom? Other people screw up drinking and get a hangover. I can die! I don't want to die, Mom, I want to live, and everything just seems so stacked against me. You think I like living like this? My childhood was destroyed by my dad's addiction. My teen years by my own. I had my early 20s taken away by an accident that was not my fault. Now my life revolves around trying to survive a faulty medical device and two blockages that almost killed me, with doctors who don't know a thing about my disease."

I tried to calm him to no avail. He just needed to let it all out, so I kept listening.

"I am not a failure! I am not a bad person! I want a life, that's all. I want to get married and have children. Do you know how hard it is in LA to find a woman who only looks at your soul and not your pocketbook? God forbid you tell them you can't drink and party. I am so lonely. Most of my friends are years ahead of me, married or graduated from school and grad school. I want that too! I love you, but I want a life of my own supporting myself, and I keep ending up in the hospital and rehabs."

"I'm so sorry, Bug. I know it has not been easy…"

He went on. "And I hate the fact you have to pay for everything."

He tried to hide his anger by looking out the window. After a few minutes, he calmed down, and I felt safe to put in my two cents. "Bug, you can have those things. I promise. We can't change the past, and you've been dealt a hard hand to play—no denying that. But if you give up trying, you lose."

Luke nodded in agreement. "So now what? Where do I go? I need a safe place to get back on my feet. I know that. I need a solid AA community. I can't do this alone…"

"How about going back to LA and that new sobriety house your friend started?"

"I don't want to cost you any more money, Mom. Don't you think I know how much I've put you in debt with my medical bills? You should be living a high life, and instead, you've just been taking care of me," he said somberly.

"Honey," I replied, "like my daddy used to say, 'If not for your kids, then for who?'"

"The sobriety house is $3000 a month, Mom.... I know you are pinching pennies paying off my medical bills that are not covered by insurance."

I replied with Grandma in my ear. "And that, my dear son, is why God created second mortgages. Before I left to pick you up, I asked Jim to start the paperwork to cover six months' rent at the sobriety house."

"I'll pay you back with my settlement money, Mom, I promise," he said, turning to me with hope in his eyes.

"My payment will be your sobriety, honey. That's all I ask," I said, taking his hand.

"Done!" he replied, smiling.

Two days later, Luke was headed back to LA. May 2 was the start of his new life at a friend's sobriety house in Los Angeles. This time sobriety was not a dream, but a dream come true.

****

The only time my anxiety was gone, or at least on pause, was when Luke was in a treatment center or sobriety house. I knew he was safe and surrounded by those who understood the game. Neurobiology is a part of addiction, and so is coming to grips with the fact that SUD is a chronic disease that demands abstinence, no matter the circumstances or social pressure. The best way to help maintain abstinence is by being with others who are in the same boat.

Back in 2012, the 12 Step program of AA/NA totally changed my son from an angry youth into a responsible young man. Even though he had more than one relapse, a normal happening for those first in treatment, the program laid the foundation for Luke's recovery. It taught him personal accountability, forgiveness for self and others, compassion, making amends for wrongs he caused to others, and being continually aware of his responsibility to humanity. Luke needed to get back on his AA program as his feeling of worthlessness was a significant trigger for relapse.

Being a part of the AA community was very important to Luke for many reasons. He knew working through the steps had saved his life by giving him the tools to forgive his past misdeeds. It also connected him to his AA brotherhood which aided in his sobriety. Being accepted in a group was vital to Luke; he was a very social person. His magnetic personality usually put him at the center of attention in any situation, and people just gravitated to him. He fed on that acceptance as it made him feel worthy and important. Being back in a house surrounded by a brotherhood solely focused on healing body, mind, and soul was imperative for Luke's recovery.

However, the one thing that concerned me about many sobriety houses was that they only dealt with substance use disorder and did not take dual diagnosis or MAT (medication-assisted treatment) into account. This was disheartening because many doctors and government agencies now considered these medical treatments the gold standard of care for opioid addiction.[6]

A significant problem is that those at the core of treatment centers still follow the science of the 1930s. That is when William G. Wilson—aka Bill W.—first published *The Big Book of Alcoholics Anonymous*. Luke had about eight copies marked up as he was religiously trying to stay the course. He had another five brand-new copies to give to new people he stumbled upon. *The Big Book* is a great tool. If spirituality and prayer were all that were needed to heal addiction, Luke would have been a poster boy for recovery. Unfortunately, SUD is a lot more complicated.

Classic AA considers the use of any mind-altering medication as detrimental to the recovery process.[7] This is an understandable concept, as during AA's early years, the mid–1930s, there was little understanding of neurobiology. However, a more balanced approach is needed as addiction science has advanced. This conundrum left Luke getting great support but archaic treatment. Dr. Andrew Rosen wrote about this in an article titled "Not All Addicts Are Alike." He said, "Brain imaging, genetic advances, and careful epidemiological research have all contributed to a more holistic systems approach to recovery. Yet, these findings have had a slow trickle-down effect on those who need proper treatment."[8]

Why is that? I wondered. It was disheartening to discover that educational standards and treatment modalities had stayed the same 25 years after I left the psychiatric hospital.

Experts were calling for change but few were listening. The *New*

York Times reported, "While most medical schools now offer some education about opioids, only about 15 of 180 American programs teach addiction. Dr. Kevin Kunz, executive vice president of the Addiction Medicine Foundation, which presses for the professionalization of the subspecialty, said, 'the content in all schools varies, ranging from one pharmacology lecture to several weeks during a third-year clinical rotation, usually in psychiatry or family medicine.'" The National Center on Addiction and Substance Abuse at Columbia University called out the medical profession's failure at every level—in medical school, residency training, continuing education, and practice—to adequately address addiction. Simply put, "the vast majority of people in need of addiction treatment do not receive anything that approximates evidence-based care."[9]

Sobriety houses are a good example. Luke had excellent experiences at them, but they were and are run by people with little formal training or educational background in addressing dual diagnosis issues. Many counselors are in recovery themselves, which means they understand the struggle but not necessarily the disease. Those without advanced clinical training tend to think everyone's disease is identical to theirs. More than that, most treatment personnel carry the "addiction counselor" or "substance-abuse counselor" credential, for which many states require little more than a high-school diploma or a GED. If one is only dealing with straight SUD, the system mainly works. If patients are dual diagnosis, they are in jeopardy. Unfortunately, people with mental illness are more likely to experience a substance use disorder than those not affected by a mental illness. According to the Substance Abuse and Mental Health Service Administration's 2021 National Survey on Drug Use and Health, approximately 9.2 million adults in the United States have a co-occurring disorder.[10]

My son was dual diagnosis. That fact was not considered early in his recovery. I knew Luke was in safe hands regarding his spiritual needs for recovery. My biggest concern was that Luke was told he only needed a commitment to the 12 Steps to maintain his sobriety, and if he couldn't maintain it, he simply didn't try hard enough and was morally defective. The problem is you can't pray away PTSD. You can't tell someone with general anxiety disorder to meditate away a panic attack or clinical depression. Imagine telling a cancer patient they have a moral defect if they can't pray their cancer away.

*****

In mid-September 2016, Luke called, telling me he felt strong enough to go out on his own again. A few men were leaving in good standing and asked him to move in with them. He called them "The Squad." I sensed from our conversation he was back on his game. At the time, I didn't realize this was the turning point in his life.

I think every parent of a child in recovery wants to try to control their kid's decisions—I mean, down to the last detail. At least I did. It gave me a sense of security—false as that may have been.

Fear lies at the bottom of that action. We all eventually face death, but for most people, no raven is perched above the chamber door calling your child's name. Like Edgar Allan Poe, you can't shoo the raven away. You just sit and endlessly bargain, trying to keep that damn bird from taking your loved one away for as long as you can.

Was five months enough time? I wondered, but that wasn't my call to make. It was hard to let go, especially under the circumstances. But if Luke was sober and trying to build a healthy life, I would help him get on his feet. Our goal was to get him out on his own.

*****

The phone rang one day. "Mom, I want to take classes and get certified as a personal trainer. I want to get my certificate in nutrition from NASM, the National Academy of Sports Medicine. I can get them both by Christmas and then get a job at a sports club and build up my client list."

"That sounds like a plan, son," I responded. "I know you'll get clients quickly. I'm proud of you. And I miss you…"

With a deep sigh, he replied, "Thanks. I miss you too. NC is so far away. Any chance you can come out for a visit?"

"Of course, Bug—I'd love to," I calmly replied. Inside I was screaming *yes* I was so glad he asked me before I started begging. By the end of the call, we had dates set and planned on a mini vacation in mid-October during my fall break.

Of all the trips Luke and I took together, this one was my most cherished.

Luke met me at the airport. From the start, I noticed something very different about him—a calm and peace I had never seen before. I could tell he had been working out again and spending time in the sun. He was also letting his hair grow out, letting go of the "have to be GQ" mode he used to live in 24/7.

We went straight to Malibu for lunch and walked the beach as he filled me in on his life. Around his neck was a seashell on a leather lanyard. Before returning to the car, he pulled a replica out of his pocket and handed it to me.

"I found these matching shells by the beach the other day and bought lanyards so we could both wear them. I have one, and now you have the other, Mom," he said as he put it around my neck. Of all those blasted gems in my jewelry box, no piece of jewelry was ever more precious than that one small shell.

After lunch, Luke drove me to a small hotel and took my rental car to an AA meeting. He clarified that attending one to two meetings daily took precedence over anything we did—that and meditation time.

For two days, we played in LA. We went to the beach, walked the Santa Monica Pier, drove up the coast with music blaring, went shopping (of course), and did some general sightseeing. He even took me to an open AA meeting. On day three, we took off to the mountains, heading for Big Bear and stopping along the way to meditate and hike a few trails.

Luke was true to his word. At Big Bear, he attended morning and evening meetings and meditated daily. Our walks around town were filled with talks about surrender and finding purpose in life that revolved around helping humanity.

It was hard to put into words my feelings as I looked at him across the table one night at dinner. A true shift had occurred. We were no longer mother and son but instead friends, two souls who connected at a deep level, grateful for the other's presence. Acting impulsively, I took his picture to preserve the moment. Of all my photos of him, this one is my favorite. It surprises people when I tell them that because it's not a glamour shot but one that genuinely captures Luke's essence. Looking at him, I felt no disease present, no ego running the show, no anxiety keeping him captive. Sitting before me was a man of integrity and grace at peace with himself and the world.

Chapter 8. Broken Policies

Luke slept in the last morning at Big Bear, allowing me time to write. My heart was heavy, knowing we would be traveling back to the mayhem of Los Angeles and going our separate ways in a few hours.

Journal entry Oct 07, 2016, 08:28 AM
A deep sadness veils a mother's heart when she sees her mothering days are at an end. It's not a sudden awareness. We know the sun will set every day, and yet we don't think about it when we are enjoying its rays on our face. But the dusk comes and cannot be denied. We yield to the inevitable and loosen our grip, holding on to a candle's flame of light that keeps the memories alive.

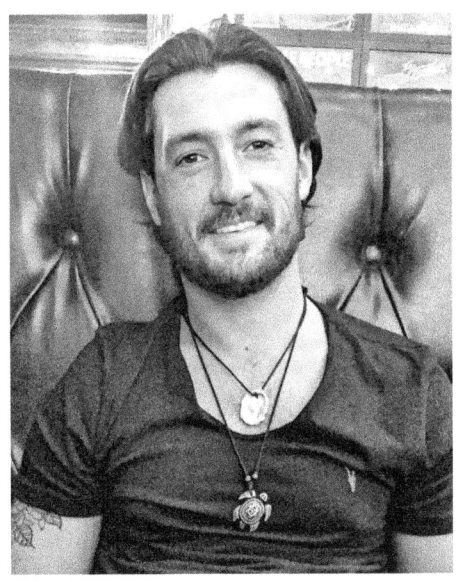

This is my favorite picture of Luke. Working hard, being at peace, California, 2016.

There is also a deep pride that swells in her heart when she sees this separate human being she helped create radiate independence, perseverance, and strength apart from her. As much as she wants to claim those traits as the dregs of her teachings, she sees her child learned despite her meddling and chuckles, "Thank God."

For some, the path to this independence was well laid out and executed, much like meticulously following the directions for a Lego structure. Others, like mine, well ... we threw away the directions long ago and merrily (sometimes frantically) started piecing together a unique craft that somehow, miraculously, turned out to be a blue-ribbon entry.

I doubt the instincts will ever go away. You know, coming to a sudden stop in the car and your arm flings across to become the seatbelt for them ... even though they are driving. Or putting in your two cents even though you are fully aware as soon as the words leave your mouth, they are more than a bit antiquated. There are also those humbling moments when you see they are smarter than you are in many areas, and you find yourself asking them for advice.

The plane will leave tomorrow morning, taking me back to my own life across a Continent's divide. I am going to have to reconstruct a life, as for the past 25 years, it has revolved around this man-child of mine. Our journey was so different than most, and here we are at the perfect place in time, building our own separate lives yet forever connected. It is time. Sadness, and yet, it is time. It is how God intended things to be. I mean, really, how else am I going to get any grandbabies?

The plane leaves tomorrow, not today. There are still memories to be made as we leave the mountains and drive back to reality. These memories will be stored in my heart-chest and keep me warm in the months to come. Sheer gratitude and grace wrap themselves around us. I will dwell on that thought to keep away the tears of sadness. Nothing can separate us from the love of God, as nothing can separate the love of a mother for her child. Not time, not age, not even the sunset of life. All is well. We are well. God is good.

When Luke drove me back to the airport, our parting was hard, but we both knew all was well in our worlds.

*****

After returning home, I saw Luke working on certifications and himself, asking deep questions and reflecting on his findings. Up until this move, Luke had been only dabbling in the arts. This was partly because I pushed him, but he had talent. His heart was not there, however. He had come to accept his place in the world. Along with that acceptance, Luke discovered a deep desire in himself to wake people up to their potential and find his own. He was a deep thinker, a man of passion and great intelligence, but he had not yet known what avenue to pursue.

Luke was also becoming my hero and inspiration. When our life blew up in 2001, it took years for me to stop feeling sorry for myself. Self-pity is a heavy mantle, and I didn't wear it gracefully. Watching Luke continually fight back made me realize I had lost only material possessions; he almost lost his life. He lived in constant pain, was disfigured, and would be in a perpetual battle with his brain chemistry for the rest of his life. As Luke fought on, he encouraged me to do the same.

With Luke working on his recovery, it was now time for me to work on mine. My stress was brought on by trying to control something that would never be in control—his disease. Time to put that pursuit away. Stress can take a terrible toll on one's health. It takes time to heal after years of trauma. For 15 years, I had been dealing with heartache, loss, addiction, and fear. Living with constant stress had taken its toll on me. Even though Luke was doing well, I had the dregs of angst locked tight in my being without knowing the consequences of ignoring it.

Chapter 8. Broken Policies

My stress hit a tipping point in late November when I sang for a memorial service. I felt a tad funny when I stood up to begin the Lord's Prayer. In the middle of the prayer, I felt the most excruciating pain strike the top of my head like an icepick. By the song's end, I was genuinely praying, not the words of the Lord's Prayer, but that God would keep me from collapsing or passing out before the final "Amen."

The pain continued, which was unfortunate as Jim and I were leaving the following day for Las Vegas to meet Luke at a multi-level marketing event. My discomfort was put on the back burner as I knew I would see my son again.

There were more than 10,000 people in attendance, along with well-known guest presenters like Tony Robbins and Richard Branson. The noise, lights, and electric environment were almost unbearable at times, causing me to walk out in search of silence. Had it just been a trip with Jim, we would not have gone, but I didn't want to ruin the experience for Luke as he was gaining ground, working to build a new life, and learning from the masters in the industry.

After the event, Luke knew he was meant to be an entrepreneur and hopefully go into politics one day, as changing public policy on drugs was not going to happen on its own. He truly felt a calling and was excited to see where it would take him. Whereas his memory was still iffy, he now felt he didn't need a college degree to be a successful advocate and entrepreneur. It was so wonderful to see a bright light burn not only in his eyes but also in his heart.

During our off hours, we went out to see the sights of Las Vegas. It's not my favorite place to visit, but we found plenty to do outside the casinos. Even though my head was still pounding, I kept a stiff upper lip as I didn't want to spoil the fun for my boys.

We always had fun as a family. I was glad Jim was finally seeing my son healthy and strong—without the drugs and the fears that once controlled his personality. Luke never thought of Jim as a second dad but as an uncle who took good care of his mom. Kind of like a "bonus dad." Jim also took great pride in caring for us both; we depended on him as our anchor.

On the last day, we said our goodbyes with hope. Luke was heading back to finish his certifications and set up his first business. I knew I had to see a doctor when I got back ASAP; besides the growing migraine, I was starting to feel little jolts throughout my body. Was it stress or something else? The tests would soon reveal it was a lot of both.

My doctor immediately sent me for an MRI and put me on anti-seizure medication. I hated how tired it made me feel, but it did stop the little jolts as the headache slowly subsided. It took two weeks of testing to find out I did not have a mini-stroke as doctors first thought when they saw little black dots on the scan. Those turned out to be salivary gland stones. Who knew, right?

On with the hunt. Early dementia was ruled out when my four-hour testing showed I was in the top third of my age and education group. Increased intracranial pressure was finally ruled out with another set of tests. Finally, the word came down from the neurologist that I had experienced non-epileptic seizures caused by moderate PTSD. I was told to slow down, retire from teaching and other outside activities that caused stress, and seek counseling.

The prognosis looked good on paper, but slowing down was easier said than done. My brain had been rewired to be constantly reactive over the years, and the stress had my processing systems in a state of chaos. It was time for some self-care.

Luke convinced me to try meditation and talk again to Tom Thompson, the town's most respected hypnotherapist and, for lack of a better word, guru. Tom taught conscious living, which includes all aspects of our lives, including the integration of body, emotions, mind, and spirit. I avoided medical doctors at this point as no pill could cure the inner turmoil trapped in my cells. Tom's hypnotherapy indeed proved to be a godsend.

*****

One step in self-care was to take a trip with family. Luke and I always tried to be together on our birthdays. In February, our business meeting in San Francisco again allowed us to meet and go to Lake Tahoe. Yarrow was now living outside San Francisco and happily agreed to come along.

The trip was an adventure, to be sure. On our way to Lake Tahoe, we got trapped between two road closings at dusk because small avalanches left us off-road in a tiny town with one hotel room available.

Chapter 8. Broken Policies

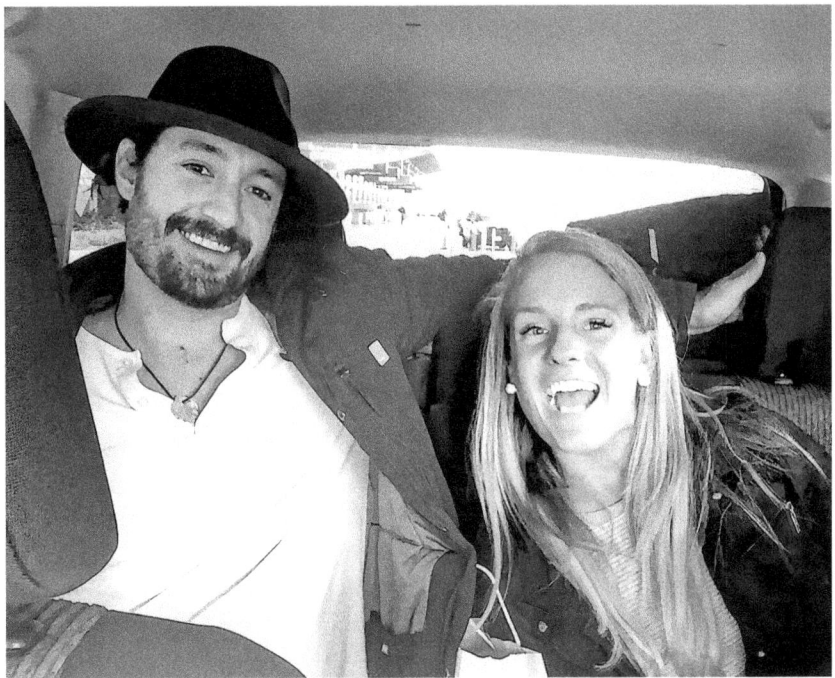

Luke's 25th birthday. Going to Lake Tahoe with forever friend Yarrow Courney.

When calamity happens, one has a choice: get frustrated or laugh and make the most of it. We chose the latter. Even though Luke and Yarrow had taken their separate paths romantically, it was evident they were still close friends and shared a deep affection for each other. I truly felt like I had my two kids in the back seat bantering playfully and keeping Jim from freaking out driving through 20-foot walls of snow.

The next morning was magical. Trying to give the kids a full day of skiing, we left the hotel before dawn. The only way to get to the next highway was via small winding roads in the middle of nowhere.

Our detour to Lake Tahoe brought us to a scenic overlook at daybreak. A raging river ran its course between the hills as a soft fog gave way to the sun. We were all mesmerized—except for Jim, who was still in military mode to get us to our destination safely. Bless his heart.

The scene was too mystical to ignore. Luke insisted we pull off so he could take it all in and meditate. I promised Jim Starbucks if he just sat tight.

I stood by the overlook, taking deep breaths to calm my racing mind. I then realized I could spend the rest of my life worrying about what might happen to Luke and lose out on the joy of our times together or stop and simply enjoy the moments with gratitude. Yes, our river was a raging one, to be sure. But to only focus on it would mean missing the colors of the morning, ever-changing in the mist. Luke was doing well today—it was time to let that fact suffice.

Luke and I sat together on a boulder in silence for a long time before he reached over to take my hand, saying, "One day at a time, Mom. Just one day at a time. Live in the moment. It's all we've got."

I nodded. "Indeed, son." I felt the stress melt away with my letting go. The rest of the trip was full of snowboarding, laughter, and another wonderful birthday dinner.

We arrived home safe and sound, thankful for another trip together as a family. Now only mundane problems occupied my mind. One was Luke's appearance. I was not crazy about his growing locks, but I had learned to choose my battles. As if it was any of my business, you know? Another concern was Luke's insistence that he and Alex would visit Costa Rica in March.

Alex was Luke's close friend and sobriety mate. Both were in discovery philosopher mode, and long hair was a part of it. So was traveling. In March, they took a week off from work and went to Costa Rica to drink good coffee, interact with a new culture, and catch a few waves. I had to laugh, knowing anyone looking at them would have a stereotypical view that they were druggies hunting a stash. In reality, Alex was finishing his Master's degree in chemistry at UCLA, and Luke was his intellectual equal. Sitting in on their conversations made my head spin as they were over my head. String Theory had not been on my reading list.

My real concern was that Luke started complaining about stomach pains, so I was hesitant for him to leave the country should another bowel obstruction present itself. The kind of care Luke would need could not be found in the far corner of the world where they were staying.

Thankfully Luke got home safe. No sooner than he returned to LA, though, his body turned on him again. Luke went to a play at Cal Arts one evening to watch a friend perform. At intermission, he got up and staggered to his car in pain. Being over 26, Luke was no longer covered under our insurance and only had Medi-Cal income-based insurance. He barely reached the ER and collapsed outside the entrance.

His friends called me the following day with the news. My first instinct was to drop everything, head out there, and be his advocate. This time Luke turned down my offer. He had The Squad there to help him. I honored his wishes. In retrospect I wished I had not.

The doctors kept Luke on an NG tube for seven days, hoping the bowel obstruction would pass on its own as before. It did not, however, and they almost let it go too long. The doctors were worried that necrosis was setting in. Luke suspected they were getting impatient with him knowing his insurance would pay pennies on the billed amount if he had the surgery. It wasn't until his life was clearly on the line that a doctor made the call to operate. Before he did, however, Luke had to sign off on a form allowing a colostomy to be performed.

All my peace was flushed down the drain in a flood of helplessness. Advocating for yourself is impossible when you're on drugs and in pain. Yes, he had good friends, but what did young men know about situations such as Luke's? I respected Luke's wishes—very reluctantly, I might add. I hoped he listened to my nagging about getting the proper anesthesia and aftercare. He was in a morphine fog once again, and his friends were loving but clueless. I knew I was on Luke's HIPPA form and called in my two cents about walking him off with Suboxone. Again, the medical staff seemed oblivious.

Right before Luke went into surgery, he was visited by a new surgeon who wanted to try fixing Luke's blockage laparoscopically before opening him back up. Once again, Luke had angels watching over him. Not only was this doctor able to fix the blockage, but he also took a laser and went all the way up and down his scar tissue from the inside, searing off any other adhesions.

With the colostomy averted, we could once again breathe. Unfortunately, the doctors released Luke two days later with a script for Tramadol, telling him he didn't need any other pain medication.

Once again, dear medical professionals—*you cannot perform surgery, give an SUD patient 10 days of morphine, and then not offer Suboxone or Methadone for a walk down.* It does not matter if one has 10 days of sobriety or 20 years. The brain has been altered and does not forget. You have lit a bio-neurological response that demands a bio-neurological solution.[11]

Yet that is precisely what happened. To make matters worse, Luke's well-meaning friends told him that just working his program and staying connected to AA would be enough. It wasn't.

I panicked. I had read too many stories of people being sober for years, even decades, who overdosed after one small slip.

One example was the gifted actor Philip Seymour Hoffman. Mimi O'Donald, his partner, shared his story in a heart-breaking *Vogue* article with Adam Green. Phillip had been off heroin for 23 years before he experienced a few stressors and slipped. Being sober and a recovering addict was, along with acting and directing, very much the focus of his life. But he was aware that just because he was clean didn't mean the addiction had gone away. His longtime therapist died of cancer, which was devastating, and he had a falling out with a bunch of his AA friends. He started having a drink or two without it seeming a big deal. Some recovering addicts say they can start drinking again after a few years of sobriety. Most in recovery say it is the devil's back door as it awakens the receptors and lowers one's resolve. Such was the case with Hoffman. A few weeks later, he was dead of a heroin overdose.[12] The world is filled with similar stories.

*****

Luke was three weeks short of his one-year sobriety anniversary before he experienced his blockage. He did not voluntarily go back on drugs but was once again forced back on them. His AA sponsor told him that having to go back on morphine in the hospital would not break his sobriety, but should he reach out and take anything to ease his cravings afterward, it would mean he would lose that year and must start over. That meant Suboxone or Methadone were not options for Luke if he wanted to maintain his status in the community.

Reading through blogs and articles, I was amazed that those in recovery, including sponsors who are not clinically trained and in recovery themselves, think cravings can exclusively be dealt with by toughing it out within the AA program. This ideology totally disregards the science that has proven "treatment with buprenorphine or methadone was associated with reductions in overdose and serious opioid-related acute care use compared with other treatments."[13][14]

Luke had terrible cravings each time he was forced back on narcotics. Then, of course, he had to detox going off them. Science tells us that cravings are a neurological reaction in the brain that seeks the substance that once eased emotional and/or physical pain.[15] Cravings cause pain. To detox, meaning to go without the substance, causes incredible physical pain.[16] Why is the use of medication so blatantly disregarded in treating SUD? Imagine breaking your leg and not being allowed to take any pain relievers, as to do so would mean you were undisciplined and weak. It made no sense!

I asked Luke once what detoxing felt like. He responded, "Image someone pours kerosene on you and lights you up. You burn. Every part of your body is on fire inside and out. You can jump in a pool [meaning using the drug] to extinguish the fire, or just stand there for days and let it slowly burn itself out as it burns you up alive."

Sometimes I crave sugar, but I have never felt that way walking away from a piece of rhubarb pie. Dr. Sal Raichbach of Ambrosia Treatment Center explains that addiction is more than just a craving or a bad habit. "A lot of people use the word craving when referring to an addict's lust for getting high, but using that word leads to a fundamental misunderstanding about the disease. The reality is that the cravings of addiction aren't the same kind of desire that someone would have for chocolate or potato chips. An addict doesn't just crave the drug; their body is functioning as if it cannot live without it."[17]

The facts remain: Suboxone and Methadone take away the fire and are much easier to walk off than opioids. Yet they are not used because the medical community is unaware and/or unwilling to take the extra training to treat "drug addicts," feeling they brought this catastrophe on themselves.

Unfortunately, most in the AA/NA community preach that they are not working the program if they do each out for MOUD. That is like telling a diabetic not to use insulin when their blood sugar escalates; if he does, he is weak. Both substance use disorder and diabetes are chronic illnesses. Both demand medical interventions, yet only one is deemed worthy of them.

Public policy is also to blame for the lack of following the science.

Only a handful of medical professionals honor the science that SUD is a disease. Consequently, it is still treated as a moral failing by policy makers. The numbers alone prove this point. In 2019, the American Diabetes Association claimed diabetes accounted for 87,647 deaths annually. In the same year, the CDC reported 70,630 documented drug overdose deaths. Both diseases have strong genetic components, are directly impacted by socio-economic factors, and are impacted by personal lifestyle choices.

Yet money is abundant for the diabetic as it is recognized as a disease. In 2015, the Special Diabetes Program created by the U.S. Congress funded $150 million per year for type 1 diabetes research. The global cost of diabetes in 2019 was $825 billion.[18]

According to a 2021 Pew Research article, "each year, opioid overdose, misuse, and dependence account for $35 billion in healthcare costs, $1.94 billion in annual hospital costs, $14.8 billion in criminal justice costs, and $92 billion in lost productivity."[19]

*****

Luke was quiet for the next few weeks, and I gave him his space. Fortunately, I had a business meeting in Napa, California, and I thought meeting up in San Francisco afterward would be nice. I knew things were not right when he stepped off the airplane. Luke was not acting high but was very thin and depressed. He never let on anything was wrong, nor did he offer information other than that he was recovering slowly.

We had a few good days doing the usual sightseeing, shopping, and eating out before we both went our separate ways. Nothing prepared me for getting a phone call five days later that Luke was in a psychiatric ward on suicide watch. Within two days, Jim and I bought one-way tickets and were on a plane for LA to be at his side and get answers.

When we arrived, we discovered that to walk himself down from the morphine, Luke started using kratom tea as his cravings were intense. Upon telling his sponsor, he was demoted back to being a "user" and felt he was no longer a part of his recovery community until he walked down off the tea. Then he could start back with a Day One sobriety chip. This rejection crushed his spirit.

He was also despondent, wondering how many more times he

must go through this intolerable blockage ordeal, which demanded his brain be relit on opioids. After his sober roommates told him he had to move out because of the tea, he drove himself up to Malibu, the place where he learned about his father's passing, and shot up with heroin. It was too much heartbreak for him to bear after he had tried so hard to put his life back together. The police found him and simply dropped him off at the address on his driver's license.

Luke had enough sense to realize what had happened and admitted himself for detox and a psych evaluation that morning. His roommates were packing up his belongings. It was up to Jim and me to figure out where his car was, drive it back, and move him out, putting his belongings in storage.

Jim and I checked into our hotel and then drove to the hospital to talk to him. With only Medi-Cal insurance, Luke was in a psychiatric hospital for the indigent and displaced. The staff was caring, but seeing schizophrenics freely roaming the halls in full psychotic states gave me cause to be concerned for Luke's safety.

Luke just wept when he saw me. "I'm so sorry, Momma, I've been trying so hard…"

"I know you have, Bug," I said through my tears. "We came to take you home."

"Thank you, Momma. I need to go home. I need to be in a safe place and get better."

"Bug, I have to ask…" Taking a deep breath, I asked him if he intentionally tried to take his life.

"I don't think so, Mom. I'm just so sad. I just wanted all the pain to stop, and drugs were the only things there for me."

I pulled him close and just held him for a long time. "We'll find another way, Luke. I promise."

Chapter 9

The Golden Years

> "If we fall, we don't need self-recrimination or blame or anger—we need a reawakening of our intention and a willingness to re-commit, to be whole-hearted once again."—Sharon Salzberg

It took a week to store Luke's belongings before we all returned home to North Carolina to regroup. The past was the past, and we agreed it would remain so. Luke shamed himself mercilessly. My heart went out to him. He had tried so hard to play by the rules that he had been forced to dance with the devil once again.

Inside I was trembling, knowing that Luke's high tolerance probably saved his life that night in Malibu. He had not yet dealt with his father's death—suppressed grief, they call it. And the PTSD from the accident was lurking as well, causing his anxiety to mount. He had reached out for pain relief which could have been fatal.

When I was stressed or grieving, I could open a bottle of wine. But my body was not allergic to wine. Luke's brain, however, was intolerant of any substance, and grief-caused pain triggered severe cravings. For him, life's time bombs, ones that hide around everyone's corner, would forever be potential death threats. Luke had a life-threatening disease and needed to find a way to deal with it. Thankfully some answers came in the summer of 2017 that proved miraculous.

During the first week home from LA, I needed to follow through on a commitment in Virginia and thought the trip could provide a good chance for Luke and me to have some fun. We packed the car and took off on the five-hour drive. Instead of putting on his favorite music, Luke asked if he could play some podcasts he had been following. Sure, why not? He seemed very excited to share them. I was expecting topics about nutrition or politics, which I dreaded.

Imagine my surprise hearing lectures from well-known college professors discussing topics like "What harsh truths do you prefer to ignore?" "Is free will real or just an illusion?" "The efficient wealth creation." "Karl Marx's German ideology." After four hours, my head spun, and I asked for a break. "Son, this material is way over my head."

He replied, "I love it, Mom! Aren't these ideas exciting?" He went on to explain many of the concepts, but I was simply too overwhelmed to keep up.

I spent two days in meetings while he was content to read in the hotel room. On the way home, he started with a whole new set of podcasts filled with more complex issues like "quantum mechanics theory" and "the fallacy of Kant's categorical imperative."

Halfway home, I paused the podcast. "Luke, you do realize these lectures are at the graduate level, don't you? Your ability to understand them—I mean, *really* understand some of these concepts here—is beyond the undergraduate level."

"Really?" He didn't know.

"Yes, really, son, really. What got you on this path?" I asked, a bit astonished at his level of comprehension.

He paused for a long time before answering. "Well … I was worried that all my friends were getting a good education, and I didn't want to be left behind and feel like a stupid fool. I figured I could learn from podcasts and listen to recorded classes online to keep up."

Dumbfounded and impressed, I replied, "Son, if you can process this type of information on your own, you have what it takes to go back to school and get a degree … or two."

Luke instantly perked up. "But what about my memory, Mom? I still have gaps and can't memorize well—I mean, short term."

"You can't remember where you parked or what you ate for breakfast, this is true, but your long-term memory seems to be fine. Especially when you hear the information instead of reading it. You are an auditory learner—like me. But we are talking about two separate yet connected cognitive processes. Critical thinking is not a matter of just collecting information. A person with a good memory and who knows a lot of facts is not necessarily good at critical thinking. I have a classroom full of them, trust me. A critical thinker can understand outcomes from what he knows and understands how to make use of information to solve problems. You cannot only understand these complex concepts but also unpack them, compare and contrast and then simplify them, which means you are excellent at critical thinking!"

Luke was again quiet before he asked, "You think I'm smart enough to go to college? I mean, I am sober now except for … you know … but I had a clean brain all last year and have learned a lot. Every night I listen to podcasts and read about philosophy, doing the assignments the professors give students. Obviously, my assignments aren't graded, but I think I am keeping up."

"Luke, I have been a college professor for years. Trust me, I wish I had your kind of mind in my classes. I know you can make good grades at a community college. You do have a documented disability and can go to student services to register, which will make it easier for you to do the work."

"I don't want a disability status and have an easier program than everyone else!" he retorted.

"That's not how it works, Luke," I told him. "The professor gets a private letter from student services saying the student needs more time for tests or special considerations like seating placements. No one knows but the professor; he or she is legally bound to keep it private. It has nothing to do with getting a free pass. You must earn your grade just like everyone else."

That night, when we got home, Luke was in his room looking at college programs in Wilmington, North Carolina, and Santa Monica Community College, close to his old neighborhood in California. His hope had returned, and he was excited to get his life back on track. My hope returned too.

*****

Luke was thin and out of shape after three months of battling depression and being unable to eat properly due to the blockage. Knowing exercise and nutrition are paramount to brain health, he built a better health routine.[1] He dug up the protocols for healing addiction and craving rehab from Dr. Daniel Amen and Dr. Charles Gant's books.

Chapter 9. The Golden Years

They are leading experts on brain health and celebrated authors who understand SUD from a bio-neurological standpoint.

Now, he was pumped, and with earbuds in place, he headed down the driveway shouting his Tony Robbins positive incantations. It was a short run, but he was ready for more upon his return.

"Mom! Can I take the car to the fitness center and get a month's pass?"

I was happy to give him my charge card. "Go for it!"

Luke was home by 1:00, totally exhausted but beaming. After a few hours in his room checking out classes, he asked if he could take a road trip the next week and look at the community college in Wilmington and at apartments. He had a whole list pulled up. We set the date for the end of the coming week.

It was wonderful to see Luke's strength returning. There was a light back in his eyes and a clear determination in each step. I was amazed at how disciplined he was in his routine. He started each day with a 30-minute meditation, took his nutritional supplements, and went on a run followed by three hours at the fitness center. At night he went to an AA meeting and found a new local sponsor who became a friend. I was exhausted just watching him.

One day I saw he was getting bored in the afternoons and had an idea. I suggested he pick up his old golf clubs in the garage and go to Knollwood, a short par three golf course down the road from our house. "Just go hit a bucket of balls and see what happens," I told him.

"I tried golfing before, Mom, remember?" he said with hesitancy. "It hurts my back, and I can't get any distance on the ball because the rods in my back limit my swing."

I simply replied, "Then change your swing, Luke. Do you remember that man out at our old golf club who only had one arm? He shot close to par, and I guarantee he had a unique swing."

A lightbulb went on above his head, and Luke took off with his old clubs in the trunk of the car. He left at 2:00. It was after 6:00 that evening when he returned, more excited than if he'd won the lottery. "I changed my swing! It took a while, but my back doesn't hurt! Man, I crushed it!"

After five days of the same routine, plus golf, Luke came home with a haircut and new golf clothes.

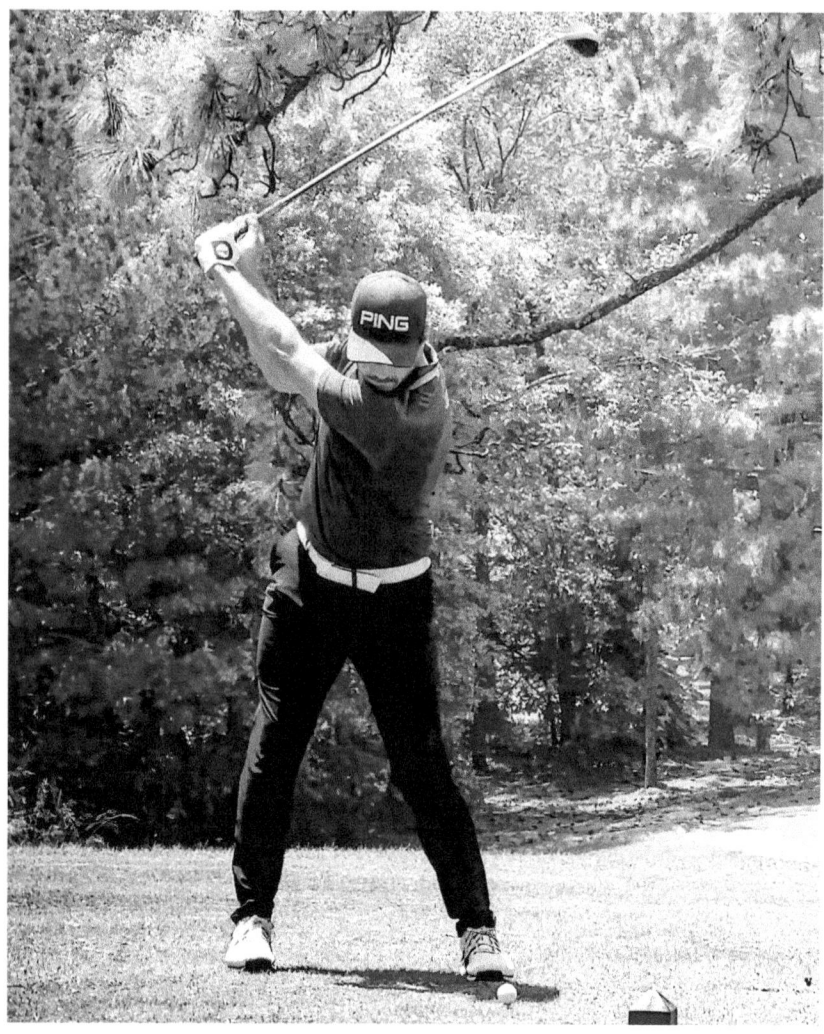

Luke changed his swing and changed his life, summer 2017.

"Hope you don't mind, Mom; I needed a few new shirts and golf shorts.." He grinned, showing me the credit card receipt. "I am really getting good—like all those years of lessons came back instantly with a few slight changes in my stance. I bet I could get even better with a new set of clubs tailored just for my new swing…"

I just laughed, telling him to get whatever he needed. My Luke was back! That week, he started a new life with golf at the center. Granted, golf was quickly becoming an obsession, but so what? Golfing gave

Luke's brain the needed endorphins to feel good again, without drugs, and that was all that mattered.

Never in my wildest dreams did I think a game could facilitate such a dramatic transition in a human being. I used to play myself, but my game was always iffy. I did shoot a birdie once. Unfortunately, it was followed by 18 strokes on the next hole, a par three. I found scoring with happy, straight, or sad faces simpler. To put my actual strokes down was just too depressing.

Luke, on the other hand, was meticulous with his scorecard. He had to be out golfing every day, and soon I had a new pastime: being his caddy. At first, I tried to play with him, but soon, I was content to ride along and watch him—I slowed down the game. It touched my heart that Luke was never embarrassed to be out golfing with his mom. As a matter of fact, he welcomed it.

Jim asked me one night if I thought golf was Luke's new addiction. "Yes. So?" I replied. I told him about a friend from the psychiatric hospital where I once worked. Carol was a drug and alcohol counselor with 30 years of sobriety under her belt. One day, after a grand rounds lecture, she was asked if being addicted to alcohol was the same as being addicted to food. She replied simply, "I've never been pulled out of a ditch with a Twinkie in my hand, I've never hid a quart of milk in the commode tank, and I've never been arrested for eating three hamburgers." Jim got my point.

The bottom line is that the brain needs the neurotransmitters dopamine, serotonin, endorphins, and oxytocin to feel good.[2] Without proper levels, depression sets in. Luke's brain was damaged due to the years of narcotics, resulting in fewer dopamine receptors than normal and a limited ability to produce the normal amount of feel-good chemicals.[3] People with severe SUD are drawn to drugs at this point not to get high but simply to feel normal. Much of the stigma of SUD comes from society not understanding this fundamental truth.

Golf made Luke feel good. The daily challenge to do better flooded his brain with neurotransmitters. Every day Luke went out trying to top his last score. Doing so lit up his brain with joy, so much so that at the end of the summer, he told me he never once thought about drugs nor had any cravings.

*****

Now, Luke was conflicted about where to live. On the one hand, all his friends in LA had family nearby; he was 3,000 miles away from his family. He admitted many times he got homesick and just wanted to be able to come home for a weekend like his buddies. On the other hand, Luke had lived in LA for six years. Many of the men there served as his support system and the LA recovery community was strong. They didn't treat each other like defective human beings and 1500 separate AA/NA meetings were offered daily. Self-esteem and support are imperative to recovery. Even though his slip counted against him in the overall AA community, many of his close sobriety friends rallied behind him as many had also slipped. I made sure Luke knew that he had time to make up his mind, even though I was secretly hoping he'd choose to stay close to home.

After playing a quick nine holes one morning, Luke took off for Wilmington to check out the community college campus, look at apartments and catch a meeting. Even though he loved me to death, he wanted a little distance. Besides, Pinehurst didn't have what he needed to create a new life as it was so low-key. I more than understood. Wilmington was only two hours away and had golf courses too. He did ask for my input on schools, as he knew that was my forte.

One of my roles as a professor was to be an advisor—not just academically but also as a personal development coach. Many of my students did not have a strong family support system or people who believed in them. Often students would come to see me just for a pep talk or to unload personal problems, looking for emotional support. Feeling confident positively impacted their feelings of self-worth, which would then translate into positive effects on their academic performance. "Momma P" they called me instead of Professor Paschal. "Alma mater," after all, means "nourishing mother."

Luke was excited about returning to school, and for the first time, I truly thought he would have a successful experience. His enthusiasm was high, but his self-confidence was low due to his two failed attempts—he needed guidance. Luke's life had been set back for six years dealing with his medical issues, impacting his core belief in himself. I could now see he needed an academic advisor and personal cheerleader to get caught up academically and emotionally. It was tricky, however, to keep my roles in their

Chapter 9. The Golden Years

separate lanes because the Mom in me always wanted to drive the bus.

After his second trip to Wilmington, Luke announced he had decided to stay in North Carolina. I was ecstatic. He said he'd found a nice loft and returned many times to attend meetings and play area golf courses. Yet I could see he was still conflicted as he hadn't put down a deposit on the loft. I was right. Luke walked into my office a few days later, stating he needed to talk to me.

"Mom, please don't feel hurt. I've been accepted back into SMCC in LA. I already have 16 credit hours from when I first moved there, plus it has a better poli-sci program than the one in Wilmington. Also, Alex just told me his roommate is moving out at the end of August and wants me to live with him. He's my sobriety anchor, and I need him in my life. Jacob wants me back, too, and I really miss the Squad. Would you be terribly upset if I moved back to LA?"

My heart sank, but I wanted what was best for Luke. "Son, I'm behind you no matter your choice," I replied.

I could see the relief in his eyes as he pulled up all the classes at Santa Monica Community College. We pored over them for the next hour, putting together a plan. I encouraged him to start slowly, only taking six to nine credit hours in subjects he liked. We set up a schedule with breaks between classes for study time three days a week, leaving two weekdays and one weekend day for working at the fitness center as a personal trainer and nutrition coach.

"Start slow, son. You will also want time to golf, even if it's just going to the driving range," I cautioned.

"Oh, of course, Mom. I've got to golf every day," he exclaimed before hitting me with a new great idea. Somehow I knew it would cost me… "Speaking of golf, Mom, would you mind if I went for my TPI level one golf trainer certificates? The classes will take a few weekends."

Luke launched into all the benefits it would offer him, how he could get clients from the fitness center, take them to the golf course for personal coaching, and so on. He always had an angle and was a great salesman.

"How perfect, Luke!" I replied. Anything to keep him connected to golf was OK by me.

Luke approached my desk and asked for a hug as if he was reading my mind. "I'll miss you too, Momma. But like your daddy once told you, the only thing that separates us is distance. You can text every day." Luke knew I needed to hear from him to calm my fears. Texting was my addiction.

I laughed. "And you better text back!" I said, holding him tight, trying to hold back a tear. "Anytime you want to come home, there will be a ticket. Besides, I like LA and will come for a visit if you want."

Luke gave me a final squeeze, then stood tall, saying firmly, "Momma, I'd like that very much. I love you, but I need to go and establish my own life."

I replied with a peaceful heart. "And that is how it should be, son. You are your own man, and you certainly don't need me anymore. This last surgery hopefully solved the blockage problems, and there is nothing more to hold you back. All I want for you is happiness and sobriety. If LA is the place to give you those things, I give you my full, undying support."

Luke replied softly, pulling me in for a hug. "I will never be able to thank you enough for all the love and support you've given me. I've got this! Please don't think I am abandoning you. You're my momma, and I will always want you in my life."

That did it. The tears flowed for us both. "Go golf!" I then shooed him out of my room so I could process in silence everything that had just happened.

The whole goal of raising children is to let them go. Luke's mishaps may have put him back seven years in his career, but surviving the traumas and working his 12 Step program had put him decades ahead in maturity. I would support him financially now as I would have had he gone to college when he was 18, and he would help calm my anxiety by staying in touch and sharing his successes. I was also touched Luke wanted me in his life. Many men walk away from their mothers, never to return.

*****

Luke headed home to LA 10 days later—new golf clubs and all. As always, I tucked a little love note in his bag and had put his name on my credit card so he wouldn't feel as if Momma was hovering over his shoulder every time he pulled it out to pay for something.

Chapter 9. The Golden Years

The summer of 2017 gave me back my son and a plethora of wonderful memories. I watched him go from a depressed man to one of hope and determination. It also helped me deal with my constant fear of losing him, which, unfortunately, is the price one pays for having a family member with SUD. People would stop me at church or around town and cautiously ask, "How's Luke doing?" With a calmer heart, I now replied, "It will always be one day at a time—but today is a very good day!"

Luke was true to his plan and had his TPI level one golf trainer certificate by October. After two months of training at the fitness center, one of his clients asked if he was a caddy. When Luke replied no, the man told him there was an opening at the famous Riviera Country Club, where he was a member, and he would be happy to call in a referral if Luke wanted the position.

Luke was ecstatic and, in three days, he had a new job. He could work his golf rounds around his class schedule and make good money in tips. To sweeten the deal, Luke could play the course on Mondays after a six-month probation period. Even though Luke kept telling me the titanium rods in his back were stronger than bone, I was naturally concerned about the weight of the golf bags he had to carry. Mothers always worry. I had to admit that Luke was in excellent physical condition and was not complaining about pain.

Christmas 2017 was a very special time to be sure. Luke finished his finals, and the Riviera gave him time off to come home and golf. Every present under the tree that year was golf related. North Carolina had unexpectedly warm weather for a few days, so naturally, we were out on a different golf course every day. I was astounded at how fast Luke's game had improved. His buddy even got him on the prestigious Pinehurst No. 2. I had to watch from the clubhouse. Dang.

That Christmas, I also witnessed a side of Luke I had never seen before—that of extreme compassion. We all were out shopping one day when the weather turned cold. Coming out of a store, we walked by a young man in a t-shirt shivering, sitting outside a store holding a sign asking for food. Luke told Jim and me to meet him in the car. From a distance I watched Luke enter a store and return with food and a warm coat. Luke sat with the young man for a few minutes. He gave Luke a

<   **Luke Paschal**   🔍

 Susan Bartz Herrick is with **Luke Paschal**.
Feb 18, 2018

Believe it or not, he is at work...

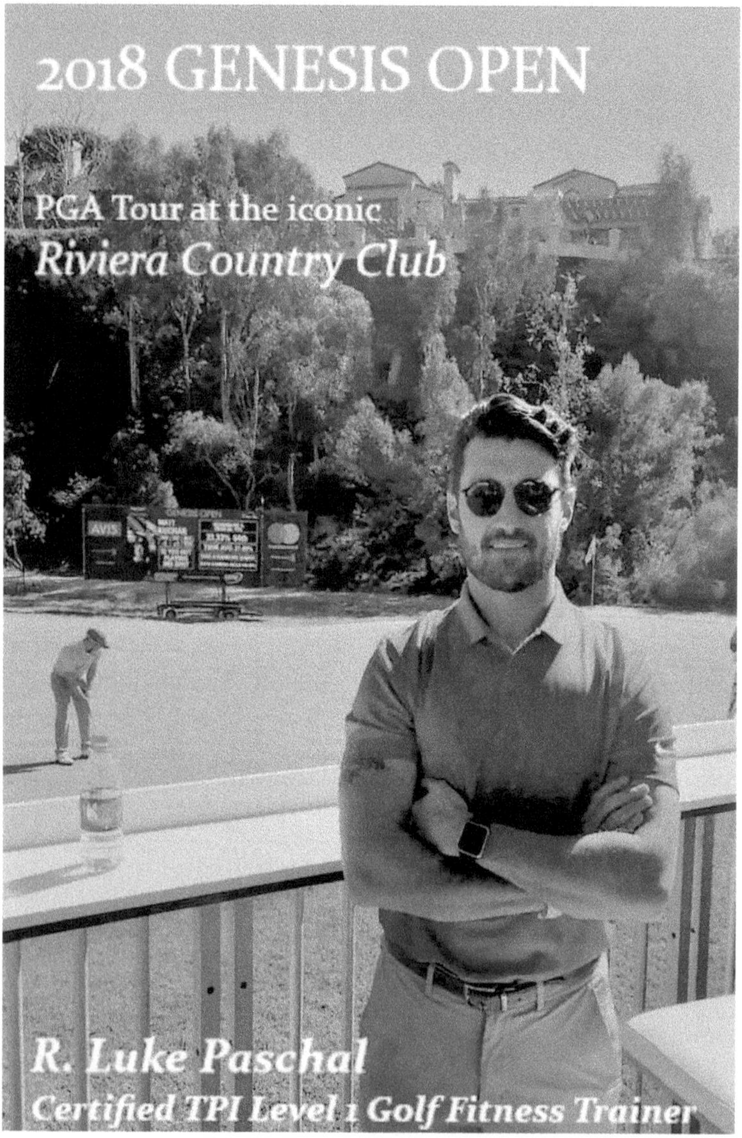

2018 GENESIS OPEN
PGA Tour at the iconic Riviera Country Club

R. Luke Paschal
Certified TPI Level 1 Golf Fitness Trainer

So proud my son is moving forward in his career.

Chapter 9. The Golden Years

hug. Luke came back to the car, saying nothing about his deed. I had tears of pride in my eyes.

Luke also gave me my most treasured Christmas present that year. Sometimes when he came home, he sang in the church choir with us. The choir was my squad—the ones who watched Luke grow up and prayed for him around the clock during his accident. They loved seeing him come back home and embraced his journey.

Our choir director asked us to sing a duet at the start of the candlelight Christmas Eve service. At first, Luke balked at the idea, but after going over it once, he decided to do it as a gift to me. His beautiful baritone blended perfectly with my voice.

That night the church was dark, with only the Christ candle in front lighting our way. We started the haunting piece "I Wonder as I Wander" from the back of the sanctuary, trading off lines and joining our voices together at the end of each stanza. With each verse, we moved closer to each other as the lyrics told the story of abounding grace. By the last verse, we faced each other with only the candle lighting our faces. Unrehearsed, we reached out our hands to each other when the song ended, then slowly walked our separate ways back into the darkness. The moment was moving, mystical, and forever etched in my heart as well as in the hearts of many who were there. The people knew us. They knew our story. They walked our journey with us. It was grace made manifest. A Christmas miracle.

*****

Back home to LA, Luke got busy and was again getting straight As in his classes, attending meetings regularly, and dating a beautiful petite blonde from Norway. Go figure. Jacob had connections in that department since his longtime girlfriend was also from Norway. I could only imagine how that quartet turned heads when they went out together.

Jacob's career in film was also taking off, landing him national commercials and a few lead roles in movies. But one night, his love life came crashing down, leaving him in a deep depression for months. He started drinking heavily and called on his best friend for help.

On our weekly phone call, I asked Luke, "So is Jacob an alcoholic too?"

"No, Mom," Luke replied. "He is only self-medicating."

"So how does one know the difference?" I asked.

Luke's answer was enlightening. "Alcohol dependency is considered a chronic mental and physical disease that can impact all areas of your life, leaving you unable to function. Remember my stupid stuff, like at Yarrow's party?" I nodded, remembering a string of painful events. He went on. "Basically, your brain craves it, and you feel you can't live without it. If you're addicted, like me, you feel worse when you stop. If you are just abusing alcohol, when you stop drinking, you feel better. Jacob was just running away from his heartbreak. He feels good now that he has stopped. His brain chemistry is not like mine. But the AA meetings are helping him regain his belief in himself, and it's helping him understand me better and why I can't join him for an occasional beer."

After our conversation, I knew I had to investigate my wine habit. Before Luke's accident, I had a glass maybe once a week. Afterward, I found myself drinking a glass or two every night. Drinking more meant I could not teach the next day as my body rebelled. But here Luke was doing well, and I was still drinking. Why?

In April 2018, we returned to Cabo San Lucas on another business training trip. My first instinct was to leave Luke in LA and not ask him to come along. Then I realized he lived two hours from the Mexico border and knew if he wanted to get drugs he would have already done so. I also reminded myself that managing his sobriety was not my place. All indications were that he was firmly committed to his program, so he met us there.

What a difference from two years ago. We had a great time, and my team was excited to see Luke strong and in control. Everyone was genuinely impressed with his recovery. He'd run in the mornings, golf in the afternoons, and meet me at the pool afterward. Luke was also building back trust, which he knew he needed to do.

But in Cabo, I realized I was the one who now needed help. I spent much time at the pool drinking wine—something I swore I would never do in front of Luke. Wine kept me from facing my demons, my PTSD.

PTSD is a sticky wicket. Georgia Hope defines it "as a disorder in which a person has difficulty recovering after experiencing or witnessing a terrifying event. The condition may last months or years, with triggers that can bring back memories of the trauma accompanied by intense emotional and physical reactions."[4] It was then I saw I had dealt with life-threatening situations and stuffed them down for more than a decade. I didn't know that was what I was doing. Everyone thought I was a woman of steel. In fact, I was living in a state of numbness, subconsciously holding back all the pent-up anguish.

No trauma can be stuffed down forever. It will manifest itself one way or another, either through disease or drama. With Luke doing well, I finally had to face my own demons.

By the winter of 2018, I had not stopped my hectic schedule. I continued piling on more than I could physically accomplish. I sat down one day and wrote out a plan of all my obligations and calculated that I needed 15 more hours a week to complete the work on my list. I was still teaching two days a week, was on the governing board of a local symphony, taught Sunday School, sang in two choirs, and wrote and directed a children's musical while trying to run a successful and demanding business. Plus, I now had a husband who was getting short-changed.

The problem was I could not stop working. My brain had gotten into the pattern of reacting to trauma using automatic response. I was being reactive to life demands instead of proactive. I could stuff down the trauma by being busy, always busy, too busy. And I found myself being short-tempered, argumentative in meetings, and all-around erratic. That was not my usual disposition.

Luke was true to his word, checking in and texting me back, but my fears of him relapsing had not abated. I continued texting him constantly. Early in his recovery, I told Luke I needed to hear from him daily. I admitted it was my obsession and that I was working on it—my core reaction was panic if he didn't get back to me in a matter of hours. I'm grateful he understood and put up with my "stalking."

My stress was also affecting my work. Lu and Janie were two symphony board members who became dear friends. One night they took me out to dinner to try to get through to me that I was overreacting to situations regarding policies. The board was split on a few issues, and I kept pushing my agenda to the point of disruption. In her usual wise but pointed manner, Lu told me straight out, "Girl, champagne corks

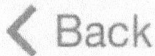

Susan
Active now • Messenger

3:07 PM

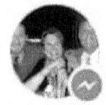 TALK TO ME

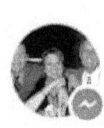 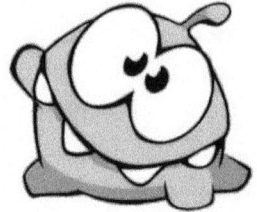

Sent from web

MOM IM AT WORK!!!

Helicopter mom on a mission.

are popping in the background, and you're hitting the deck as if it was shrapnel. What is going on?"

I didn't know. I just knew I could not stop. I recognized my friends were trying to help me and heeded their words. "I need to step down from the board, ladies. I can't see the forest for the trees, and I'm not doing anyone any good."

They encouraged me to stay on and felt they needed my expertise, but with a split board, I knew I was right and it was necessary to let go to let peace reign. They understood and thankfully remain close confidants.

To make my life more complicated, there had been a complete change of personnel at church. With new people came new ideas, and I was a part of the old guard. In my saner days, I would have let matters

Chapter 9. The Golden Years

go and stepped back gracefully. I did not this time; in short order, I was distanced from the place that had once saved my life. I was shattered, abandoned, and left feeling betrayed, so much so that I talked Jim into putting our Azalea Street home in Southern Pines on the market and started planning to move back to Fayetteville. Financially it was a good move, so he agreed. He could also see I needed a change and was helpless to comfort me.

The migraines came back also, as did the little jolts. One afternoon at 4 I reached for the bottle of wine, stopped in my tracks, and asked myself *why*? Numb. I just wanted to be numb. Wine made me numb, and I didn't have to face my trauma. *This had to stop!*

I sought out a PTSD therapist and started dealing with my issues. Soon I saw my pain did not happen overnight, nor could it be stopped overnight. It would be a long road back, and I prayed for the strength to walk it. My doctor also put me back on an anti-seizure and migraine medication. Again, it helped, but the side effects made me very tired and, unbeknownst to me, slowly induced a chemical depression. The drug also reduced my need to drink, and I stopped cold turkey, leaving me to face my heartaches without liquid anesthesia.

*****

I was thankful when Luke called one day, pulling me out of my funk. The topic de jour was his girlfriend. It made me feel good that he trusted me as a confidant. Instantly I could tell his heart was troubled. He informed me they got along great, but he wanted a committed relationship. She was only 21, however, and just wanted a fun, part-time boyfriend. Luke felt used and that she was just playing him until he'd had enough. And she drank excessively one night, making a fool of herself—he knew he could not be with anyone who abused substances.

"I broke up with her, Mom. I did it for me. I deserve someone who wants the same things and respects me and my program. But it hurts."

I told him how proud I was of his strength to do what was best for him. "What you did takes courage, Luke. Are you handling it OK?" I was afraid this heartache might be a trigger for him to reach out to his past habits.

"I'm OK. I'm on the phone with my sponsor a lot," he laughed before getting to the nitty gritty. "I am lonely, though. Alex spends most of his time in the lab or at his girlfriend's place. I mean, I am busy with school and work, but it's hard to come home to an empty place every night."

We talked for more than an hour that afternoon, sharing heartaches, trying to help each other cope. I encouraged Luke to stick to his guns and reassured him the right woman would one day cross his path. Luke, in turn, helped me work out a few AA steps, numbers 7 and 6 in particular: make a searching and fearless moral inventory of ourselves and admit to God, to ourselves, and to another human being the exact nature of our wrongs and shortcomings. He was so helpful, and I again stood amazed at his maturity and insights. He helped me see I had been blaming the world for problems I helped create. Then he taught me step 7. I needed to change my attitude, which would permit me, with humility as my guide, to move out from myself toward others and toward God. He was so right.

At the end of our conversation, I remembered a significant upcoming event. "Hey, Bug, you've got an anniversary coming up, right?"

"Yes, I do. June 2 marks year one of my sobriety. I will speak at our meeting, and I'll get my one-year chip and the traditional cake." He hesitated before asking in an earnest tone, "I know you are busy … but could you come out here for the celebration and stay for a while? Alex is not home much, and you can stay on the sofa. It's comfy."

"I'd love to! Is 10 days too much?" I blurted out.

"Perfect! Two weeks if you can manage," he replied. Three days later, I was on a nonstop flight to LA with Jim's blessing.

Luke picked me up from the airport and promptly drove me to the beach. He had bought a used SUV large enough for his surfboard and was anxious to show off his skills. He looked so happy and healthy. I just took in the surf from the beach and let the crashing waves push away my stress.

That evening Luke took me to the meeting where he and a few others were presented their one-year sobriety chips and cake. Much to my surprise, he spoke of his journey and acknowledged me for being his anchor in the storm. We both had tears in our eyes as the room gave him a standing ovation. All the years of disappointments were washed away that night. I could see Luke had overcome odds that would take most people down. He was rising like a phoenix out of the ashes. The man had so much courage. So much fortitude. I could see how others reacted to him and that he was well respected and dearly loved. A graduation ceremony from college could not have made me prouder of my son than watching him receive his chip.

Afterward, we strolled the shops in Santa Monica. Luke talked me into buying him a new hoodie, then promptly took his old one off and gave it to a homeless man on the street. He told me he promised himself that for every new item of clothing acquired, he would give one of his old ones away to someone who needed it more than he did. We ate, and he bought extra burgers for those in need hovering outside—hoping I didn't mind. Of course I didn't.

I realized that night I only knew who Luke was when he was at home in North Carolina and honestly had no idea what his life was like every day in LA. He had gone from a hurt and angry boy who used drugs to mask his pain to a man of substance and compassion because he transmuted that pain into power. Luke knew what it was like to be frightened. He took it upon himself to practice *noblesse oblige*—the responsibility of privileged people to act with generosity and nobility toward those less privileged.

*****

Luke and I also took the time to go and see his attorney, Ricki Parker, who lived in Santa Barbara. Negotiations started with Luke's lawsuit against the maker of the failed IVC filter, and she wanted to prepare us for what would happen during the deposition.

Until then, Luke and Ricki had only spoken on the phone or exchanged emails. We agreed to meet for an informal lunch at her house to get acquainted so she could hear Luke's story firsthand. At the end of the afternoon, Ricki saw how much Luke's life had been forever altered by his surgery and was touched by the closeness Luke and I shared. As a mother herself, she understood our bond. Yet Ricki was also tough as nails. Representing hundreds of others' personal injury cases had brought out the Momma Bear in her. She felt optimistic about Luke's case because of the mandatory reintroduction to opioids and his subsequent surgeries. She also stood in awe of his fortitude to soldier on.

Luke was excited. He saw he might be able to recoup his life, get caught up monetarily with his friends, and be totally independent of me stepping in and helping with rent or other goodies—like new golf clubs. The mood soon changed when Ricki told him the opposition would argue to discredit him as a former "drug addict."

I protested. "Ricki, chemical dependency was the price Luke paid for his life!" I then recapped our experiences with the opioid debacle within the medical community at the time of his accident. "He was doing fine until he had to undergo that horrific surgery to get that filter out."

"Susan," Ricki replied, "I more than get it. My own niece got hooked on the stuff while battling breast cancer. When she went into remission, no one would help her get off the opioids, acting as if the addiction was her fault. The medical community left her high and dry with us, trying to figure out how to save her from the problem it had created. Trust me, I understand what you are going through."

"I can hold my own, Ricki," responded Luke.

Ricki's 30 years in practice gave her just cause to counsel him. "Son," she said, "you don't know how vicious they will be trying to destroy you. Unfortunately, in most courts, once the word 'drug addict' is mentioned, the jury may turn against you. They don't understand it is a disease. You'll just be a junkie dressed up in a suit in their eyes. You just need to keep up the good work. The more years of sobriety you have behind you, the harder it will be for them to discredit you. Therefore, I suggest we not go to court but settle to avoid you losing everything because of the stigma of addiction. Only if that's what you want. It is your call."

"You said years, Ricki," I chimed in. "It's already been three since his surgery. How much longer can this go on?"

"They will try to take it to infinity, hoping people die or just give up. I suspect another two years before the court sets a deadline."

Luke had been counting on that settlement money. Now, he put it on the back burner. Luke told her, "Whatever happens, happens, Ricki. I know who I am and what I stand for. We'll just take it as it comes, and I will go on living my life. Money can't buy peace of mind, and I won't let the fear of losing it take away mine."

We drove home feeling good about the situation. Luke felt confident he had picked the right attorney, and I knew he no longer depended on the settlement for a good life but was leaning on himself and the spiritual path he found through AA.

For the next 10 days, Luke would do his usual schedule allowing me to nap on the sofa and read. It was a much-needed respite and a good time for some self-care, giving me time to reevaluate my life. My son had become my hero. If he could forge on after what he went through, so could I.

We had so much fun those two weeks. Every evening Luke came home excited, with great ideas for new dining experiences. Korean BBQ was our favorite, and he knew the perfect place. In his free time, we went sightseeing, driving down the Pacific Coast Highway, listening to his favorite music, or golfing. In the evenings, we'd return to his place and sit back, talking or watching documentaries in front of the fire. Never once did I think of drinking a glass of wine.

When it was time for me to go home, Luke told me the Riviera was closing in July to rework some of the greens and asked if I'd mind if he came back to North Carolina to play golf. Naturally, I was excited knowing I could ride along in the cart. Besides, I had a gift for him in the making. When he got back seemed the perfect time to spring it on him.

*****

In 2014, Jim and I bought a lot at a prominent golf club in Pinehurst called Forest Creek. We had been searching for some time as our plan when we got married was to sell our separate homes and build a home together where we could enjoy retirement.

The Pinehurst area offers more than 40 golf courses, so it was not unusual for anyone to live at a golf club even if they didn't play golf. We joined as social members; I loved the pool and Jim played tennis. Besides, the real estate market was down then, and we scored a golf course lot for half its original price. It was too good of an investment to pass up.

The two golf courses were designed by Tom Fazio and ranked in the top 200 residential courses by *Golfweek* magazine. Jim and I were drawn to Forest Creek for its quiet atmosphere and the winding paths that encompassed the property. We weren't savvy to its prominence in the golf world. Luke did know, however, and was thrilled when we told him. Growing up, he would drive by Forest Creek drooling, dreaming of the day he might be invited to play at least one round there.

As chance would have it, the founder of Forest Creek, Terry Brown, was also a symphony board member. Over the years, we became good friends. One day at lunch, Terry announced that Forest Creek would soon offer a junior membership. My ears perked up as the initiation fee was much less than the regular membership. It was based on a sliding scale that would increase yearly until the junior member turned 40. Applicants had to be approved and sponsored by a member who could vouch for them.

Over the years, our family had many dinners together, and Terry knew Luke to be a good man. For that reason, Terry offered to sponsor Luke if he was interested. I instantly took him up on his offer. I knew Luke would be thrilled beyond measure to be a member. Plus, I knew Luke was making enough as a caddy to pay the monthly dues. I could recoup the initiation fee in time. And yes, I did have an ulterior motive. Luke would be home more often.

The first morning he was home, I called Luke into my office and presented him with the keys to his locker.

"You bought me a junior membership at Forest Creek? *Mom!* Are you kidding me?!" he exclaimed as if he had just won the lottery.

"You have earned it, Luke," I told him. "Life has presented you with some incredible challenges. Most people would become bitter, blame God, and cave into anger or resentment. You did not. With each painful encounter, you chose to move forward in defiance of your setbacks.

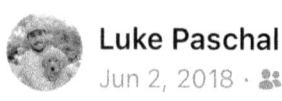

Luke Paschal
Jun 2, 2018

One year.

"Fall down seven times, stand up eight."

His work continues. "One day at a time."

You are my hero, and I am so very proud of you. Happy one year anniversary, Bug. Now, go golf at your new club!"

"You want to come along, Mom?" he asked, as we usually golfed together.

"No, son. This is your day. Go meet your pro, set up your locker, and establish yourself."

Luke grabbed the keys and took off. Eight hours later, he came home exhausted. He played all 36 holes. But he was glowing as he told me, "When I walked in, they all called me 'Mr. Paschal.' God, that felt good! They treated me like an equal."

"You are, son," I replied. "You are the only one who needs to accept that fact."

*****

Luke returned to LA on a golfing high and connected with a friend who became a constant golfing buddy. Nick and Luke met at the driving range and hit it off instantly. They played almost daily and were very competitive, enhancing both their games.

Alex had just graduated from UCLA and was headed to Cornell on a full scholarship for his doctorate in chemistry. I knew their friendship would continue via the phone, but that meant Alex's room was now vacant. Soon Luke called to tell me he had found a new sober-living roommate named Chris.

Chris and a woman named Tammy had been dating for a while, but she took one look at Luke and it was all over. Luke felt uncomfortable about her overt flirting when she visited Chris. Finally, he brought it to Chris' attention one night after Tammy left.

"You can have her, Luke," Chris said with indifference. "She goes through men like water through a sieve."

"You sure you don't mind, man?" Luke asked, a bit surprised.

Chris gave him a wry grin and said, "Good luck."

Thus, the romance began. Luke was not looking to get serious; he just wanted some company. He was flattered by Tammy's puppy dog adoration and relieved she was also in sobriety. Alcohol was her demon. After years of pageants in the Dallas–Fort Worth area, she had fallen into the trap of medicating her loneliness with champagne. It didn't hurt that she was drop-dead gorgeous with an oil tycoon father and a socialite mother. Though divorced, they wanted the best for their daughter and sent her to Los Angeles to become a movie star.

I thought nothing of the relationship at first. When Luke started dating a woman he really liked, I'd usually get an exuberant phone call with all the exciting details. The phone call about Tammy was much different. After an hour of catching up on classes and golf, he simply said, "Oh, I'm seeing someone."

"A pretty, petite blonde?" was my usual reply, suspecting he was trying to find another woman like Yarrow.

"Of course!" We both laughed. He then told me his golf scores of the day before we hung up.

Our calls were getting shorter and shorter, but I didn't mind. After Luke's long lonely spell that spring, I was happy he was connecting with new sober friends and off making a life for himself once again.

In October, I received an odd text. "Hey, Mom. Guess where I am?" After countless wrong attempts, I found out he had hopped a plane to Iceland to help a travel blogger friend with her equipment on assignment. The pictures he sent were breathtaking.

"New girlfriend?" I asked.

"No," he replied. "Truly, she's just an old friend. Can't seem to get Tammy to understand that I'm not cheating on her, but I couldn't turn down the opportunity. The plane tickets were only $350, and I could stay in a room for free. I am caught up in my classes, and the Riviera gave me the days off."

"You've only been dating Tammy for a month, Luke…"

"I know. Don't worry about it, Mom. She's young."

"How young?" I replied, remembering the last girlfriends.

"Twenty-three…" he replied cautiously.

There are times mothers speak their minds and times they need to keep their mouths shut. My inner voice told me to butt out.

"Be safe, honey, and enjoy your trip. And bring me home a nice Icelandic Christmas present!" I said as I signed off.

"It's already in my bag. Love you. Bye," Luke replied with a smile in his voice.

*****

Chapter 9. The Golden Years

Christmas is not a great time to move, but the truck came on December 18, the same day Luke flew home. To avoid getting in everyone's way, Luke and I took off from the airport to Washington, D.C., leaving Jim to direct traffic with the movers.

Washington was cold and magical. Luke and I began our visit with his favorite Smithsonian stop, the National Air and Space Museum. His father had taken him as a boy, bringing back good memories. Naturally, he went on all the flight simulators, and I got a personal tour guide who knew all the aircraft and its history.

Luke was a fun travel companion, always making me laugh, especially when he would take off on any given subject in one of his many accents. Arnold Schwarzenegger was my favorite. He drew quite a crowd one day, bringing a modern art exhibit to life.

The kid was blessed with incredible humor, a quick wit, and a magnetic personality. He used those skills to charm everyone and basically was just a person everyone loved to be around. Someone once told him he'd make a great stand-up comedian, but he balked at the idea, feeling it would be too invasive of his personal life. Plus, he had loftier ambitions.

"I want to live here in D.C. one day, Mom. It feels like home. I could do a lot of good for people. I understand their pain," he said pensively as we stood in front of the Capitol.

"Go for it, Luke. Follow that calling," I encouraged him.

"I've got a plan," he said as he winked at me.

Luke and I drove home, once again listening to captivating podcasts on various topics. My niece Jenni drove in the next day, and Luke took off to Worth's house so we girls could decorate the tree. He came home later and grilled us steaks and made his famous mashed "taters" and asparagus. I thought three tomahawk steaks were a bit much, but we managed to finish them. The dogs had a feast too.

Late that night, Luke and I sat in front of the fire for a cup of hot cocoa and a long talk. I could see he had changed so much this past year, but he felt he was still so far behind his contemporaries. He also struggled with feelings of inadequacy.

We sat in silence for the longest time before he spoke. "Mom, I see Worth, Jacob, and Alex and all they have done. Sometimes I fear I don't have what it takes to have the same good life."

"Luke, you must remember Worth is 20 years older than you are, Jacob is not in recovery, and Alex wasn't almost killed in an accident followed by multiple surgeries. Do they treat you like the black sheep?" I asked.

"No. Not at all," he replied quickly.

"Then the only one making you feel inferior is you, and it's up to you to turn that around. Those men have their journey, and you have yours. The main thing is they love and respect you. That makes me feel good knowing that you will have family and friends here for you one day when I am gone."

"You're not sick, are you, Mom?" he asked seriously.

"No, Bug, but I am getting older. Sixty-three does not feel as good as 43 did. My blood pressure is a bit high sometimes, but I am taking care of myself. I'm not going anywhere, son. I'm having too much fun being your mom. Besides, I want grandbabies," I laughed, trying to calm his concern.

Luke got pensive and said quietly, "I can't wait to have a family of my own, Mom…"

"What about Tammy? Is she the one?" I asked tentatively.

"No. I mean, she's all right, and I must admit I love her fawning all over me. Did you see the cashmere sweaters she bought me for Christmas?"

"I did. Quite pricey, kid."

"Her family is wealthy, Mom. She's an only child and a trust-fund baby."

"You do seem to attract the heiresses, Luke." I poked the bear. "What is this, number three?"

Luke just glared defensively at me before answering. "I met her family, and I really like them. Her dad reminds me so much of Dad. Same Southern style and sense of humor. He is a very successful businessman with many connections. Her mom is a doll and likes me too."

"Mmm." I nodded apologetically. "Just make sure you are with Tammy because you like her, son—don't get sucked in by the glitz."

"I'm not," he responded. "Truthfully, I have a plan, Mom."

"So what are you going to do?" I asked, trying to get the Christmas spirit to return.

"Buy a puppy!" he exclaimed.

"You are not serious! Puppies take time … money … and…"

Luke was up the stairs before I could finish.

*****

The next day Luke flew back home to Los Angeles. Two thousand nineteen was a brand-new year, one filled with opportunities and the potential for success. He had plans in his back pocket and wasted no time putting them in place.

The first plan executed was getting a Golden Retriever puppy. He so wanted a dog like his Katie, slow, calm, sleeping all day and snuggling at night. What he found was a bundle of love on steroids. He called to share the good news.

"You didn't!" I sighed.

"Yup. She loves me. Her name is Ellie Mae. I have a crate, toys, and all the stuff a puppy needs."

"You have everything but time to raise a puppy," I chided.

Luke hated it when I was right. In three weeks, he called, shaken and upset. "Mom, I've been asked to move or give up Ellie Mae. She barks non-stop when I am gone. I take her out in the mornings before I leave for school and always spend time with her when I get back, but she needs 24/7 attention and pitches a fit when I leave."

In genuine sympathy, I told him, "I'm so sorry, honey. You truly don't have time for a puppy. Why not do the noble thing and find Ellie Mae a good home?"

"No!" he cried out. "She's mine!" He then pleaded, "Will you and Jim raise her for me?"

I had no problem taking Ellie Mae, but I knew Jim would have reservations. We had just adopted a long-haired German Shepherd puppy named Max. He was seven months older than Ellie and coming into his maturity. Two unneutered puppies of different sexes could prove a challenging mix.

"Listen, Luke, I'll ask Jim and get back to you, but I doubt he will agree. Taking care of the dogs is his role around here."

"OK," he sighed. "Please, Mom. *Please*?" I could hear the pain in his voice.

I sat Jim down and explained the situation. I was right. He was reluctant. I asked him to call our vet and ask about the timing for fixing one of them. Much to my delight, the vet told us Ellie would not be able to have puppies until she started her first cycle in a few months. When that time came, she could get spayed, and there would be no problem. After hearing the expert, Jim reluctantly agreed. He knew training two puppies would be a handful. But he was a true dog whisperer at heart.

I called Luke with the news. "You do understand, son, she will always be your dog, but Max, Lucky, and Ellie Mae will bond into a pack after she is here for a while. Separating them will be devastating to them all. This will be her home."

"I know, Mom," he responded sadly. "Make sure she doesn't forget me, OK?"

"I know she won't. You were her first daddy—they never forget," I reassured him.

Luke had all her papers in order two weeks later and bought an airline crate ticket to send Ellie Mae to North Carolina. Surrendering his girl to us was perhaps the hardest lesson he had to learn—letting someone go in their best interests, even if it broke your heart.

To ease his pain, Luke threw himself into his work. He was a popular caddy at the Riviera. His ability to read not only the game but also the players made him in constant demand for individual rounds and for the tours that came through. He was featured on a Farmers Insurance Open social media post. Many famous Hollywood producers and actors asked for him by name. It was obvious that being a caddy was a means to an end for him, and they enjoyed the intelligent conversations that came with his expertise. I so enjoyed getting the texts updating me on his encounters.

Luke had another surprise for me. I knew he had been getting excellent grades and was planning to continue his education at a university. UCLA was the obvious choice since it had a reciprocity program with the California community college system. He had other ideas.

"Mom, I've applied to the University of Pennsylvania," he announced on a call one day.

I choked. Luke had talked about Ivy League schools' special programs for some time. They are online programs specially designed for older students who had unusual and challenging circumstances out of high school but have proven themselves in the ensuing years. To be fully admitted, Luke would have to prove himself through their gateway program by passing five classes with a 3.0 GPA or better. Still, I knew getting into the Bachelor of Applied Arts and Sciences (BAAS) program was a long shot. He was smart enough; I was very concerned about his previous academic history.

"Mom, if I don't apply, I'll never know, right?" he said with determination. I just shook my head, knowing he'd be disappointed.

Three weeks later, Luke called me, ecstatic. "Guess what, Mom? I was accepted!"

"Dang, son," I replied in a mild state of shock.

"I know, right? Can we go for a visit in May? I want to meet my advisor and get my ID card in person."

"Absolutely!" I replied, amazed. Never underestimate the power of perseverance.

*****

Luke was off and running. He had already gotten a taste of free enterprise by running his own small Shaklee business. Now he was trying to find a link between his desire to change policy for those suffering from SUD and his desire to start his own company. One day it all came together in the most unlikely place—the golf course.

Luke was out golfing with his buddy Nick when they got to talking about how CBD oil helped Luke's back pain and regulated his anxiety. Nick was skeptical at first. Luke filled him in.

In 2018 a U.S. farm bill legalized CBD products, removing them from the Controlled Substances Act. CBD is one of many compounds in the cannabis plant. Two of the compounds in marijuana are THC and CBD. These compounds have different effects. THC is the best-known compound in cannabis. It has a psychological effect that creates a mind-altering "high."[5]

CBD, in contrast, is not psychoactive. It does not change a person's state of mind when he uses it. However, it may produce significant changes in the body, showing some significant medical benefits, including the ability to reduce anxiety, enhance cognition, help with movement disorders, and reduce pain.[6] Luke needed this natural product to help him cope without the harsh side effects of pharmaceuticals. Even though clinical research supporting these findings wasn't published until 2019, Luke had heard by word of mouth that CDB oil was effective for regulating pain and was taking it regularly. It was legal to buy CBD in California.

Luke did his research and told Nick about an article he found on Financialnewsmedia.com. It claimed the Brightfield Group, a cannabis industry company, estimated the CBD industry's value would reach $22 billion by 2022; that didn't include any products with THC.[7] Luke wanted a piece of that pie. He knew it would take time to work through the individual state laws but bet he could start his own company in California, building it up enough to be able to expand as the rest of the country caught up.

By the end of 18 holes, it was decided they would create their own CBD company—Arrow Organics. Nick would take care of the paperwork, and Luke would be the front man, designing the website and marketing the product. It was a perfect match according to their skills and personalities.

So many junk CBD products were already floating around. Luke knew he'd have to try to verify his product through independent testing facilities. Each batch that came out had its results posted on the website. Luke was insistent their product would be natural, safe, and effective and would follow the strict guidelines of quality he learned from dealing with Shaklee's quality assurance program.[8] He'd use only certified organic hemp and get Alex, an expert chemist, to help create the formulation.

Nick and Luke filled the orders from Luke's apartment for the first few months. The kitchen was turned into an assembly line: bottles were filled, labeled, sealed and shipped. After a few months, the workload was consuming too much of their time, so Luke hired the production out to a company which allowed him to spend time marketing. In no time, word-of-mouth recommendations, along with Luke's local marketing skills, made Arrow Organics a hit, and orders started pouring in.

Luke was more than busy in the spring. He put SMCC on hold and dug into his online classes at U Penn. I was still pinching myself that he got accepted.

Luke passed his first two classes with grades in the high 90s. He would send me his grades on individual assignments and the

Chapter 9. The Golden Years 211

professors' commentary. "Very impressive work!" "Excellent commentary." "Have you considered going into public policy, Luke?" All the feedback enhanced his confidence.

Luke learned to work with his memory challenges and ADD by effectively multitasking during this time. I was more than impressed by Luke's learning system; it was unique. He turned a small closet in his room into his office with a TV-sized monitor to project his research holding his attention while working on his large-screen computer.

Instead of celebrating Easter at home that year, we met at Penn so he could tour the campus, meet his advisor, and get his picture ID card in person. I spent an obnoxious amount of money in the bookstore buying sweatshirts and other Penn paraphernalia, still pinching myself. Who would have thought this kid who once couldn't sit still and had brain damage could be so successful?

Luke's appointment with his advisor was at 3 p.m. I walked the campus for more than an hour, waiting for him to finish. Over dinner, he spilled the beans.

"I found out today why I was accepted, Mom—at least part of the

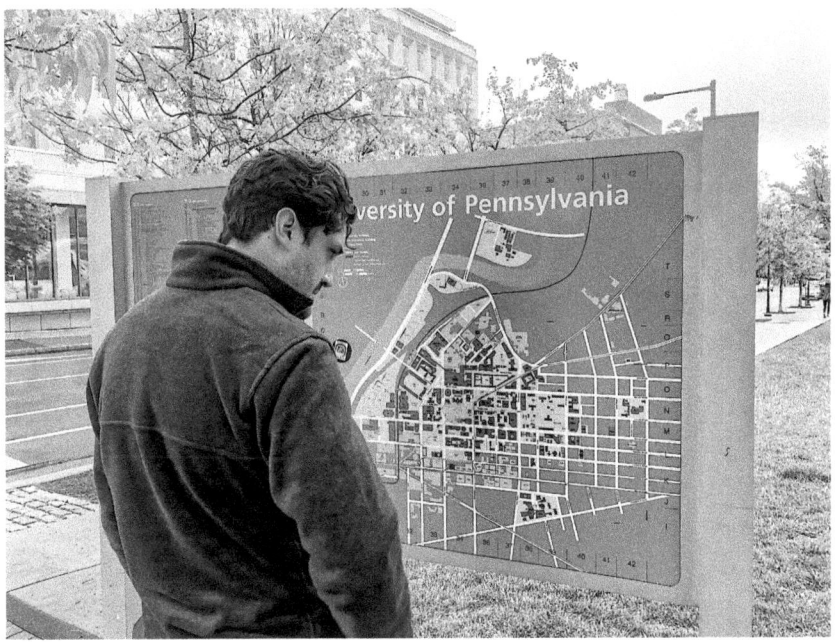

Luke finding his way at the University of Pennsylvania, 2019.

reason," he said with a smile. "My advisor once worked as a drug and alcohol counselor. She knows the misinformation about the disease and wanted to allow me to get back what I had lost. Apparently, my story touched her—that was my entrance essay. I promised her I would use my degree to advance the cause."

"That's wonderful, Luke," I replied.

"She hugged me when I left and congratulated me on my grades from the spring term. I know I can do this, Mom," he said with renewed determination. "I think the universe is giving me hints to move back to the East Coast."

"Just take it one day at a time, son. The doors will open for you when the time is right."

Chapter 10

The Perfect Storm

> "Meteorologists see perfect in strange things, and the meshing of three completely independent weather systems to form a hundred-year event is one of them. My God, thought Case, this is the perfect storm."—Sebastian Junger

In February 2010, we managed to get together in Carmel, California, for Luke's 29th birthday. Tammy came along but was a bit put off that we didn't stay at the Ritz. Her lavish lifestyle concerned me as I knew down the line, she would expect Luke to provide for her in the manner to which she was accustomed. Even when she visited the previous year, Tammy wouldn't stay at our large home on a lake. Baxter's golden rule was in full effect—he who has the gold rules. Luke was constantly making excuses for her immature attitude. Once again, I said nothing as I wanted the trip to be memorable. I hoped in time Luke would see that Tammy growing up with every want and whim paid for was not a great recipe for internal growth and spiritual development.

One month later, the world shut down with Covid 19. I was particularly concerned for Luke's health. He no longer had a spleen, the organ that supports immune health. His lungs had also been severely damaged in the accident, putting him in the high-risk category. Over the years, he had painfully fought off a plethora of other viruses, so naturally, Covid deeply concerned me. Yet because of how California law was applied, Luke was not eligible for the vaccine when it first came out.

LA was getting very restrictive, so Tammy's father generously flew them in his Gulfstream to stay at the Texas ranch. They had the ranch to themselves for one month, along with the housekeeper and the grounds staff. Tammy's mother was holed up in her high-rise condo in Dallas, and her father was living with his girlfriend du jour in his penthouse at the Ritz.

One afternoon I got a phone call from Luke. "Mind if I come home, Mom? Things are getting a bit tense here. And besides, I miss you."

"Sure. You know I'd love that," I replied. "Do you feel safe flying commercially?"

"Tammy's dad is having his pilot fly me home," he replied. "We've gotten to be good friends. He even lets me take over the controls every now and then."

"Well, I can't argue with that," I replied, knowing how passionate Luke was about aviation. After all, he had been flying flight simulator computer programs since he was eight.

"Great!" he replied. "See you in a few hours. I'll text you from the air before we land at Pinehurst."

It was so good to have Luke back home. After a nice dinner, he filled me in on the details outside by the lake.

"So what's up with Tammy?" I asked. "All not so good in paradise?"

"It's never been paradise, Mom. You have no idea how often I have tried to break up with her," he blurted out.

"I've always wondered, son. She is obviously in love with you. You obviously are not in love with her," I said, glad to have an open-heart conversation again.

"I love her. I really do…"

"But…"

"Mom, when Tammy was drinking heavily after high school, she got disowned by her parents and became a high-class escort to survive."

"Oh," I replied in genuine surprise. "You mean just an escort or…?" I tried to draw him out, but he didn't bite.

"After a while, she hit bottom, and her parents sent her to a recovery house in LA. They took her back under the condition she stayed sober. She's got three years now. But she still seems to have a 'men' fetish. Chris warned me, but I didn't care."

"I remember you telling me about her dating Chris when you first met her," I said.

He turned his glance downward.

"What I didn't tell you is that before she was with Chris, she hooked up with just about every guy in AA," he said with some disdain. "Tammy has a past, and I'm not sure I can get over it."

Well, I wasn't expecting that one. Yet I felt the need to add some perspective. "Luke, pretty much everyone, especially those in recovery, has a past they'd like to forget. Does she know about *your* past?"

He thought hard for a moment, remembering his active use days. "You've got a point, Mom." We both nodded. "It's more than her sleeping around. I know she's been faithful to me. She's trying. We both have our flaws, but we also have different life goals. She is so sweet, but I can't talk to her about anything that really interests me."

"You have Alex for that. You know, honey, not many people can keep up with you. String Theory and all…"

"I know. But all Tammy talks about is Hollywood and fashion. I'd like a professional woman who wants to partner with me in the political arena. She wants the Hollywood life and to hobnob with celebrities. She also wants to become a runway model." He sighed.

"Luke, she's only five-two."

"Oh, I know. Doesn't seem to faze her."

"Tammy wants the Kardashian life, then?"

"Yup. And with Daddy's help, I am sure she can pull it off. But I am so done with the material demands LA makes on people. I want to go to law school in the East. Public policy is so important to me. After doing so well in my classes, I know I could get through."

"I think it's the only way to get changes made regarding SUD, Luke. I know you would make a great congressman," I replied in full support.

"Thanks, Mom. I do too. Tammy just laughs at the idea." He paused, then continued. "She also wants me to work in management at her father's oil refineries after we get married. He'll set up a satellite here."

"You'll be a bird in a gilded cage, Luke," I gently warned.

He nodded in agreement.

"So why don't you just break up with her? Is it the money?"

He was silent.

*****

Luke was glad to be home. North Carolina was much less restrictive than California. The golf courses were open, and restaurants were open with limited indoor capacities. Churches were in lockdown but not the malls. Luke was even allowed the Covid vaccine due to his missing spleen, which made us both feel better.

Our family made the best of a bad situation and tried to keep busy without tripping over one another. Jenni escaped to our home with her canine entourage consisting of two noisy Chi-Chis and a Boxer mix. Thankfully they all got along with our pack. She and I got pretty good at making sourdough bread from scratch. Luke golfed and took the opportunity to take flying lessons from an old family friend. Poor Jim had his hands full with the seven dogs. For excitement, we'd send the troops out to find toilet paper. But that was our only real challenge in surviving the lockdowns.

Yet life had changed for us all. I finished the semester with less than half my students in class online before fully retiring at the term's end. Jenni lost her job due to downsizing. Luke had to put university classes on hold for financial reasons as his place of employment closed for a few months. However, Luke reregistered at Santa Monica

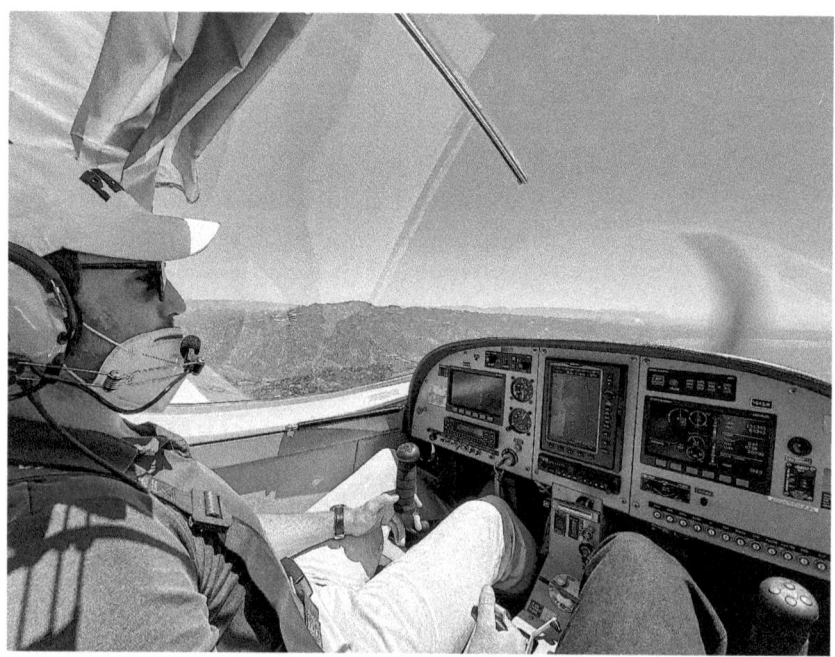

Luke had goals. Here he is logging hours for his private pilot license.

Community College to finish his associate's degree one. He was assured those classes would be accepted as transfer credits when he returned to Penn.

By the end of May, everyone had decided it was time to return to their respective homes and try to live their lives navigating the mayhem caused by Covid. Before Luke returned to LA, we celebrated his third year of sobriety. This time I made the cake.

*****

Luke's father had been an experienced pilot and he had told us numerous times that it was rare for only one incident to cause an airplane to crash. A good pilot could glide down with an engine failure, fly around in bad weather, make a navigational error and recover, or survive a mechanical malfunction. But when two or more incidents happen simultaneously, the plane is in grave danger of going down. Unfortunately, that is what was happening to Luke. One by one, the stressors were taking a toll on his brain chemistry and overall mental health.

Tammy's father sent a plane to Pinehurst to pick up Luke and take him and Tammy back to LA. Her reception of me on the tarmac was cool, yet she ran into Luke's arms with great affection. I didn't care. I only wanted him safe.

In October, Luke took another break to come home to golf. I could tell he needed to get out of LA once again. This time he flew commercial.

We spent most of those days on the golf course, allowing him to share his frustrations. In California, AA meetings were shut down. They could not even be held at the beach, only online, leaving no time for socialization and personal support. People were breaking their sobriety left and right. The overdose numbers were climbing, but no one seemed to care. Golf courses were closed, restricting Luke from getting the needed endorphins he received from playing his daily rounds. Classes were only online, again restricting socialization. Restaurants were take-out only, leaving him trapped in his room. He also could not go out to market Arrow Organics and sales were falling off. He was falling into a deep depression. I understood but sensed something else was bothering him, but I didn't pry. One night he totally broke down after a phone call from Tammy.

"I'm so mad at her, Mom," he raged, trying to hold back tears. "I wasn't going to tell you, but it hurts so bad, and I need advice."

I assumed Luke broke things off, but that was not the case. We grabbed some iced tea and went to the backyard with Ellie Mae.

"Tammy broke into my phone when we got back to LA. She was sure I was seeing someone in Pinehurst. I wasn't! But she went back through years of texts and found some rather ugly ones I wrote to friends about her when we first met."

"Ouch," I said quietly.

"I know, right? She broke into my phone!" he shouted.

"No, I meant ouch for her. That must have hurt," I replied, reminding him of his actions.

"Mom, those texts were almost two years old! I can't trust her," he said, trying to defend his position.

"And now she can't trust you?"

"That's what she says. But I know there is something else going on. I just can't put my finger on it."

"So you broke up?"

"Not really. We're just going on as 'friends with benefits,'" he said sadly.

"I will never understand that type of relationship, Luke…"

"No matter." He ignored my statement. "I have done everything I can to make it up to her. I've apologized. I tried to make amends. I come over when she calls, then she sends me home. I fill her car, and she won't answer the door, telling me to drop her keys in the slot. She says she's forgiven me but is acting so cold."

I just nodded, letting him get it all out. We were quiet for a long time before he went on. "Mom, I think I have fallen in love with her after all. And now she doesn't love me anymore. I am so broken."

Luke choked back his emotions while I gave him space to process. After a while, I told him about the Japanese art form of kintsugi, where broken vases are put back together with gold connecting the broken seams.

"I've known many couples who have hurt each other through affairs and managed to put their marriages back together, making it more beautiful than before."

"You think she might forgive me, Mom?" Luke asked in desperation.

"Listen, Bug, if the relationship is strong, you both will recover. If your relationship is what I think it is, it won't."

"What do you think is really going on?" he said, pulling himself back together. "The truth will be helpful here, Mom. Don't sugarcoat it."

"OK, then. Son, I've suspected for a long time that Tammy is a love addict. You said early on she has had a string of men. She falls in love, and the chase is on. It is all about the 'feeling.' The problem is the 'feeling' is not love. The correct term is 'limerence.' It's a chemical reaction built into us all for procreation. It gives us a 'high' feeling, producing a big dopamine dump. But once the chase ends and she gets the guy, the 'feeling' stops, and she moves on, thinking she's not 'in love' anymore.[1] It's a typical reaction of a girl emotionally abandoned by her parents, especially her father."

"She is a daddy's girl, to be sure. And you're right. Her father has never spent more than a day or two with her since she's been a little girl," he replied. I could tell it was a hard truth to swallow.

"Tammy has been chasing you for 18 months, Luke. You were her cocaine. You kept the limerence feeling alive as you were emotionally unavailable. Trust me, I know. That's why I could stay with your dad for 13 years. We were married, but he wasn't emotionally invested, which kept me chasing his attention."

"I always wondered. I'm sorry. I guess you do know what you are talking about."

"I do, Luke," I responded, returning to my memories.

This situation was all too familiar. My daddy loved me very much but was always too busy to spend time with me. I lived for his infrequent affection. Waiting for it created "the feeling." It is no wonder I had chased Baxter. Much to my surprise, he started chasing me after I left him, telling me how much he loved me. *Love doesn't choose an airplane over their family,* echoed in my head. Yes, I did understand what was going on with my son. Another family curse. This one was on me.

Knowing I had hurt Luke's feelings, I tried to lighten the mood by saying, "I want you happy above all else, Bug. I will accept any woman you choose if she makes you happy. Please know that fact."

"I do, Mom. Thank you. We both screwed up. I guess what I did was just as emotionally immature as what she did."

I agreed, happy to see he accepted his part in the debacle yet went on to prepare him for what might be coming down the pike.

"The tables are turned now, Luke. That is why she is playing games. Now that you are chasing her back, she may not want you anymore. It appears Tammy lost interest and, therefore, 'the feeling.' She's also afraid to be alone—thus the friends with benefits. I bet you anything she's on a dating website as we speak, looking for someone else, and is just stringing you along until she finds a new man. It's classic behavior." I said cautiously.

"She is not!" he shouted at me. "She'd never do that."

But that is precisely what was going on.

*****

After thinking things through, Luke realized he never truly loved Tammy. He cared for her deeply and considered her a true friend who had been there for him as he rebuilt his life. For that, Luke was grateful. But mostly, he loved the security she represented. His doubt he could have a wealthy life on his own kept him tied to her. He was ashamed to be so weak. I assured him it was a life lesson his old mother had learned decades earlier.

Upon returning to LA, Luke took some flowers to Tammy's condo to make amends, as their last conversation had been very unpleasant. He wanted to end the relationship with some dignity. Unfortunately, Tammy threw the flowers back at him, announcing, "I only accept flowers from florists, not from Fresh Market!" as she slammed the door in his face.

Frustrated, he returned to his car, slamming his fist on the steering wheel. His hand ricocheted off down to the shifter, shattering the side of his hand. He called me from the hospital and sent the x-rays in a text.

"I'm OK, mom. Just pissed off." He said, still irritated.

"Did they give you narcotics for the pain?" I tentatively asked.

"Yes. No. I mean, the doctor offered them to me, but I declined. It hurts like hell, but that's not the worse part."

What could be worse? I thought to myself. Luke said, "I can't play golf for eight weeks until it heals, and the break will probably leave a calcium deposit changing my grip."

Chapter 10. The Perfect Storm

"I am so sorry, Bug. About Tammy too. I know that must have hurt."

"It did, but at least I saw firsthand what my gut told me all along. I'd always be her puppet on a string, and I am worth more than that," he said with firm resolve. "Oh, and you were right. When I returned to LA, one of my AA buddies told me she was on a dating app only for the rich and famous. She's been on it for months."

"I am so sorry, Bug," I replied as we ended the call. Sometimes you hate to be right.

I hurt for my son, as would any mother. I knew it would take time for his broken heart to heal, but I worried more about his growing isolation without a girlfriend. Break-ups are huge stressors that cause so many people to relapse. Moreover, I was worried about his broken hand, which had unforeseen repercussions. Without golf, Luke's endorphins would decrease. Our texting became an hourly event. Slowly I saw a clinical depression setting in.

The pressure of his upcoming deposition for his IVC filter ramped up his anxiety. He went to a doctor who prescribed Clonazepam, an anti-anxiety medication, and Clonidine, a blood pressure medication. Both drugs can have severe side effects. For Luke, they were worsening his depression. For the first time in three years, I became concerned about his sobriety. I could tell the medications slowed his thinking, and he was not his usual energetic self. Up to this point, CBD oil had seemed to keep things in check. These were not ordinary times.

*****

Luke's long-awaited deposition was scheduled for the week of Thanksgiving. As expected, the IVC filter attorney went after Luke with a vengeance, bringing up his past drug use as he placed a picture of Luke's dying father on the Zoom screen. The deposition went on for seven hours. Luke was shaken and could not remember details, which frustrated the interrogator.

The attorney finally blasted Luke, "Why do you keep saying you can't remember?" to which Luke replied, "Because I was in a coma and on life support. Go ask my mother."

Three days later, I was served to testify in late January. Bring it on.

Luke came home for Christmas depressed and worried. He

thought he'd blown his testimony. He planned to use his settlement for continuing his education and thought he was watching all his dreams dissipate into thin air. Thankfully he started dating an attorney online, which perked up his spirits. A petite blonde, of course.

Meanwhile, it was my turn with the IVC filter attorney back in North Carolina. My preparation for the deposition was surprisingly devastating. Until now, I had managed to suppress all the memories of Luke's accident, surgeries, and relapses. The numb state that had kept all those feelings locked away for more than a decade took over. Returning to the trauma memories took the lid off my emotional Pandora's box, leaving all the demons taunting me.

The first night I opened the CaringBridge website to reread my posts, I immediately closed it, shaking uncontrollably. It truly hit me that I almost lost my son. All during that time, I was in an actual state of shock. Now I had to face reality head on and dig through all the medical files going point by point over Luke's devastating injuries.

After calming down, I called Rebecca and asked her to go through the 18 injuries listed on Luke's hospital admittance paperwork. Her response was not what I expected.

"Susan, any one of these injuries should have killed Luke. It's a medical miracle that he survived. I would have given him no chance at survival if I had seen this chart that night. Just answer the questions you can, and if you don't remember, or don't know, leave it at that. There is no point in me breaking down a miracle."

Deposition day finally came, and I was shaking like a leaf. Zoom on.

Round one began. The first two hours focused on Luke's injuries. Then the attorney tried to persuade me that I agreed to the filter. I did not. His late father signed the papers.

"Well, how convenient," snipped the attorney. "You are his mother and must have given your approval!"

"No, sir," I replied calmly.

He pushed on. "You mean you had no idea what they would do? How could that be?"

I fired back, "Because my son was fighting for his life. All I could focus on was my son and the machine breathing for him. The journal entry from CaringBridge even states I had no idea what any of the

Chapter 10. The Perfect Storm

medical procedures were for, including the IVC filter." End of discussion followed by a break.

Round two. I was interrogated about Luke's drug use. "Is it not true he was a drug addict before he had the filter?" the attorney asked with a smirk.

"He was chemically dependent, sir," I answered, maintaining my poise. "Severe SUD is the price we paid for his life after the accident. It's the cross we must bear, but we do so gratefully as he is still with me today. He's had many years of sobriety since and is getting excellent grades at the University of Pennsylvania."

He looked taken aback for a second before pounding on. "But he abused drugs again after his stay in the treatment center after the surgery, did he not?"

My not-so-calm reply spewed forth with vengeance. "The number of narcotics used to keep him alive was obscene. After the treatment center, he had three other intestinal blockages that required going back on them. No insurance for detox. You gutted my child and expected that experience not to cause additional trauma?" The attorney quickly called for a break, and the screen went dark.

Round three. The attorney's demeanor changed. He was quite nice, trying to trip me up on previous answers, but to no avail. Then, out of the blue, came the attack. "Ma'am, do you know how many lives these filters save annually? How many millions of people are alive today because of them? And here you are, trying to tell me they're a death trap?" he railed confidently, playing his ace card.

That did it. This calm, composed mother, dressed primly in pink, took off after him in a red rage. "Sir, millions of people get on airplanes that careen across the country daily. They go up, and they come down. For them, it was a good day. But every once in a while, people get on an airplane that has a mechanical failure. They go up but come down in a fiery crash. For them, it was not a good day. Luke was on that flight, metaphorically speaking. One of your filters had a mechanical failure, almost killing my son." Dead silence. End of deposition.

Our attorney negotiated a large settlement for Luke three weeks later—much higher than anticipated. I collapsed in tears. Luke could finally relax, knowing he was now financially secure.

*****

Soon after my deposition Luke called to tell me he had been rear-ended coming home from Yarrow's house. They had always kept in touch as she was his go-to girl in times of crisis. Minimal damage was done to his car, but he had whiplash. His auto insurance paid for him to see an orthopedic specialist at UCLA.

The news was not good. Luke's back had been compromised. The screws at the top of his implant had cracked his vertebra tab. They were now encroaching on his spinal cord, explaining the growing numbness in his left arm and the back pain.

To make matters worse, caddying—carrying two heavy bags daily—was causing his upper back to curve forward, moving the other top screw closer to his spinal cord. Bottom line, Luke's back apparatus was starting to fail, just as the neurosurgeon in Florida had warned could happen back in 2010 after his accident.

Surgery was recommended, but the doctor warned there was a possibility he could be paralyzed if the surgery was unsuccessful. Should he choose not to have the surgery, he would continue to bend forward, which could also eventually cause him to be paralyzed. Once again, Luke was facing a Catch-22 situation.

"What are you going to do, son?" I asked with dread when he called with the report.

"I'm screwed, Mom—totally screwed. My health insurance won't pay for this surgeon, and I can't have just anyone do it. I need a real specialist. I guess I'll just have to wait until the settlement money comes in and buy better insurance," he replied grimly.

"You cannot caddy anymore, Luke!" I cried out.

"I will only use a cart. I promise," he said, trying to calm me.

"What about your pain?" I asked in desperation, knowing he would once again be placed on narcotics.

"I'm dealing with it. Please don't worry, Mom," was all he said before hanging up.

Why God? Why does he have to go through surgery again? Why can't my son get a break?! I screamed to the empty room. Numbness took over again. I knew what was coming—that he'd have to dance with the devil again. I just prayed he could once again rise to the occasion in his warrior mode. God help us both.

By mid-winter, Luke and I started texting multiple times daily and calling every few days "just to chat." He knew I needed reassurance that he was doing OK. But Luke was also afraid about me dying from Covid as my heart had started to give me problems. In March, I had an elective outpatient procedure that was almost canceled midstream when my blood pressure soared to 200/110 for more than 30 minutes before the surgical team got it under control. I wore a heart monitor for two weeks, and it was discovered I had a heart murmur and was put on blood pressure medication. After losing his dad, Luke was apprehensive about losing me too.

I could also tell he was lonely and feared he was clinically depressed because he could not exercise or play golf. Luke stopped dating after the attorney he had been seeing started stalking him. The new girlfriend didn't want children, so that relationship ended. He was also getting fed up with LA in general and was beginning to make serious plans to move to the East Coast. He told me he went to the mountains to take a break from the city but knew that for now his entire focus was on finishing his associate's degree. We made plans for him to spend the summer at home in North Carolina to sort out the rest of his life.

In mid-March, I got concerned when Luke complained his night terrors were back and he could not sleep more than three to four hours a night. That had happened when he was a kid. *But at age 30?*

Then, in the middle of the night, I got a frantic text telling me about a vivid nightmare about evil forces fighting for his life. He was panicked, convinced he would die. I instantly called him. We talked about the dream for more than an hour. I tried to unpack the stress in his life that was subconsciously dictating the nightmare. To better calm him down, we made plans to go to Washington, D.C., to look for apartments in the spring. That night he saw his time in LA was indeed coming to an end. It was a good thing.

*****

Easter was perfect in Southern Pines. Luke arrived tired but excited about coming home and moving back to East Coast permanently. But he had low energy and didn't play much golf. His hand was still bothering him. Thankfully, the settlement was done, and he could begin planning how to invest so he could return to school full-time in the fall.

Still operating under Covid restrictions, our church conducted its Easter Sunday service outside under a tent. Fully masked, I sat back from the choir chairs, admiring my two handsome men. Later we had a delightful yet "interesting" brunch with friends at Forest Creek Golf Club. Two ladies at our table had very different political opinions. Luke was sitting between them. We all heard the delicate volley of words bounce across the table and held our breaths. Out of the blue, Luke skillfully defused the situation with a cleverly worded political parody as he changed the subject. The kid was good. He was already a great politician!

We took off for Washington, D.C., to scout apartments the next day. The streets were empty, and the hotel held an eerie Covid void. Very few stores or exhibits were open, except the International Spy Museum, which gave us a fun outing. Mostly we looked at spacious apartments in the Navy Yard area and took a tour of Georgetown. Luke was looking at a political science program there that would give him more options than the Penn liberal arts program.

That night I made a yearly budget template for Luke to fill out, showing him how far his settlement would go (or wouldn't go) should he choose this high-living lifestyle in D.C. while attending school full-time. Hmmph. Nothing like a reality check. Maybe he'd look at Raleigh this summer when he came home.

When I dropped Luke off at the airport, I tucked a long letter in his bag encouraging him to close his chapter in LA with gratitude and thank those who had helped him on his journey. We gave each other the usual long goodbye hugs even though I knew I'd be seeing him in a few weeks. His attitude was good; he knew the settlement check would come soon after all his medical liens were settled.

I did notice that Luke was distracted when he got back to LA and a bit out of sorts. His texts kept talking about his depression. I shrugged it off. *Who wasn't depressed during the pandemic?* Yet I counted the days until June when he would be home and I could once again relax.

On the morning of May 28, I received a text from my good friend Marcia. Our close bond had evolved over the years around praying for our two children who suffered from mental health disorders. Whereas I had freedom with Luke's SUD, Marcia was homebound, keeping her eye on her chronically depressed, schizophrenic daughter Kelly.

Chapter 10. The Perfect Storm

Reading the text, I sat stunned, reading her unsettlingly calm message that Kelly had just committed suicide. The police found her in her hotel room. I knew Kelly had gone for a visit to New York City, telling her mother she wanted to get back to her favorite place where she once worked as an architect. We both assumed her schizophrenia was under control with the medication she was on. Marcia never suspected that Kelly's voices had called her there to end the pain once and for all.

Kelly's death hit home with a devastating punch. Instantly, I wanted Luke to come home. I feared the isolation in California would be just as detrimental to him as it had been to Kelly in New York. It had just been in the news that many in the AA community were caving in to their stressors. The CDC noted that during Covid, there were more than 78,000 drug overdose deaths in the United States, an increase of 28.5 percent from the previous year.[2] In LA, it was even worse—a 48 percent increase during the first five months of the pandemic.[3]

I called Luke with the news. It hit him hard. He and Kelly were friends and had gone to Interlochen together. We talked for hours that day about the destruction Covid was leaving in its wake, holding each other in grief over the phone.

*****

My inner voice told me something was terribly wrong. My instincts were right. On June 3, I received a letter from Luke confirming my fears about his depression. He wrote:

Dear Momma,

Just to start things off, this is NOT a suicide email. I would never take my own life, but you need know the whole truth about what is going on with me, as I don't know what to do. I am miserable. I have held this from you because of your blood pressure and overall health. Every single day I am miserable, barely able to do functioning daily tasks, and it stretches past depression.

Back when I was with Tammy, she started drinking with her friends after years of sobriety as she wanted everything to be normal and to go out with people and not be that weird couple that doesn't drink. I am ashamed to admit one night I decided to join her as many of our friends in recovery started drinking also. Unfortunately, I lost the greatest thing I ever had, and that was my sobriety. I stopped soon afterward and reworked my steps.

The pressures started to mount with the upcoming deposition in November, so I went to a psychiatrist who prescribed clonazepam, and I have been taking it since.

Going back to LA after Christmas was hard. Our AA meetings online were just not the same as in person. We could not even meet at the beach. The golf courses were closed, and rounds at the Riviera were almost nonexistent, putting me on federal assistance and unable to golf. I felt I blew the deposition because they attacked me so hard for being a drug addict when in fact, up to that point, I had almost 3 ½ years of sobriety. It was more than I could take. I fell mom and reached out taking a synthetic opioid from someone I knew.

That's when I went to the mountains to try to detox because I couldn't study taking drugs, yet I can't function without them. I am in pain! When the doctor told me that one of the screws in my back was touching my spinal cord and that I could be paralyzed with or without surgery, I crashed. How can I possibly go through another surgery? He put me on an antidepressant which made me feel like crap and ramped up my anxiety.

I know this is hard to read, but please know the only thing I want is help. I have been weening myself down and down from everything, but in this process comes incredible depression. I have nowhere to turn. I hide in my room because I don't want to go outside. I am still the man I want to be. I just can't believe I let this happen. I hate this life. It is filled with darkness. Darkness that will not go away, and I don't know how to fix it.

I had thought about withdrawing from all of my classes and going into a real detox where I can have a clean head and begin to build myself back up, but my insurance only covers indigent places or where they send guys from prison. But nothing can be done until I do that. But I can't afford to lose this semester. I am stuck here in this saddened position, not knowing what to do, and it killed me not to tell you this, but it is the truth.

I don't have any desire except to be free of all mind-altering substances. I just want to be free. I have to be free, so I can rebuild and have hope again. I went to see an addictionologist who gave me suboxone. But I couldn't even stop for the 3 days to get on the suboxone. I have a bottle of it that he gave me, plus some other meds from him to help me detox.

So will you help me? I have weened things down enough that I could possibly finish my detox with you at home. It would be a really hard few weeks if you are willing to take care of me. It has killed me not telling you this, as I would love nothing more than to be celebrating my 4th year of sobriety. I lost it. I lost my time, but now I can't stay sober by myself long enough to get days because I am so lonely and cannot do schoolwork detoxing. That's why I decided to take the summer off from school.

I love you so much, momma, and I know reading this hurts you. But nothing serious has occurred, no arrests, no massive destruction of self, nothing permanent. All of my hopes and dreams have dissipated because of this. All I want is to be sober again. I will do anything it takes to do that. I just need your support and help to accomplish this because I am backed into a corner I've never felt before. Please, I hope you still love me and look at this as a slip so we find solutions as to how to deal with this. I love you so so so so much. Please look at this with love and not fear. I'm not a 22-year-old who wants to drink with the ladies and get high to feel better. I am trapped. Stuck in this cycle that has to break, or I will go insane of loneliness or whatever these chemicals are doing to my brain. I can get through this and be the love and joy you once knew. But it has to start with me going through a detox to clear my head.

I love you, Luke

How could I have been so blind not to see his torment? Instantly I called him. "Of course, I will help you! *Come home!*"

*****

Luke arrived on June 6 after finishing his classes and thus all the requirements for his associate's degree. We agreed he would taper down his medications and begin his detox in a week. Luke gave them to me for safekeeping with a daily medication schedule. I begged him to let me take out a loan for him to go to a good treatment center, but he refused, telling me he would only allow me to pay out of pocket for a PTSD specialist and a psychiatrist to monitor his progress. He was convinced his settlement would come any day, and if he could not get off by himself, he could go into treatment for as long as needed.

On June 12, we went together to Kelly's memorial service. We were shaken. Luke and I sang the praise songs together, holding hands and crying when Marcia spoke of Kelly's struggles. When she saw Luke in the receiving line, Marcia grabbed him, saying, "Take care of yourself, Luke." They hugged for a long time, rocking back and forth in sorrow.

On our way out to the car, I begged Luke, "Promise me you'll never put me through that, Bug." He never took his eyes off the ground, answering quietly, "I'll try not to, Momma."

When Luke stopped taking the drugs, the detox began. It was brutal. Every inch of his body was on fire, relentlessly consuming his brain, making him cry out in agony. For days he stayed in his room sweating and shaking. I had to change drenched sheets twice a day. One afternoon I could not find him. Calling his name, I heard a moan from my darkened bedroom. There he was, in my bed.

"I'm sorry," he whispered softly. "It smells like you…"

Heartbroken, I crawled next to him, kissing his forehead and stroking his sweaty hair. "It's OK, honey. I'm here. You're going to be OK."

Luke had Suboxone with him but refused to take it. He had been brainwashed into believing that using it was not being true to the AA/NA program. Maybe some people don't need it, but after all the drugs from surgeries and personal use, I knew he was not one of those people. I begged him to reconsider. He stayed true to his program.

After 10 days, Luke slowly started coming back to life. He excitedly told me about the AA meetings over Zoom and all the support he was getting from his friends. The meetings ended two weeks later when Luke had to go back on Suboxone—the cravings were just too intense. He was deeply disappointed. I was not.

"I'm glad you are taking care of yourself, honey. I'm also sorry the Squad does not understand you may need to be on Suboxone to maintain your sobriety," I said, again angry at their resistance to following the science.

Both Luke and I were convinced he could bounce back the same way he did in 2017. Unfortunately, his body was not rebounding as it once had. He joined a fitness center but could not stick with going for long, as he was riddled with back pain. He tried running but came home walking, out of breath and complaining of stomach pains. He went golfing almost daily but could barely make it through 18 holes due to losing stamina. To make matters worse, he was disappointed that a calcium deposit developed over the break in his hand, changing his grip. He was no longer a scratch golfer.

Trying to offer support, I set Luke up with an old colleague of mine for medical intervention. Because addiction was not his specialty, the doctor never took the class hours required to prescribe Suboxone and, in Luke's case, refill it. All he could do was offer the antidepressant Bupropion. Unfortunately, in a matter of three days, it ramped up his anxiety so much he had to abandon it. Finally, Luke was put back on Clonazepam to bring the anxiety down. The deadly game of pharmaceutical chess was on again, and I was concerned that Luke's game pieces were falling off the board.

Even though Luke put on a brave face, I could tell something was bothering him at a deep level. There was a quiet desperation settling in. Thankfully he was not holed up in his room as was his usual way of coping with depression. Instead, he was downstairs with me messing up the kitchen and watching off-the-wall documentaries while eating his epicurean creations.

One sweltering afternoon the heat kept us in the house watching documentaries on mushrooms. For years Luke and Alex had been fascinated by the mycelium of below-ground fungi, aka mushrooms, and how they connect the world underground. So it didn't surprise me that Luke was hunting out alternative substances like psychedelic mushrooms to cure depression and SUD. Between documentaries, he showed me a recent Johns Hopkins study on its psychiatry and behavioral science website that showed the mushroom psilocybin, given with supportive psychotherapy, produced rapid and significant reductions in depressive symptoms. Most participants showed improvement and half achieved remission through the four-week follow-up.[4]

Luke also pulled out more articles about lysergic acid diethylamide (LSD) and MDMA (3,4-methylenedioxy-methamphetamine). It was thought they could treat mental health disorders and addiction, generally with the close guidance of a psychiatrist or psychotherapist.[5] Needless to say, I was very skeptical as, in my youth, LSD was for tripping hippies at Woodstock. Luke reminded me that LSD research started in the 1950s but the drug was abused and then banned since it was not regulated.

"A classic Big Pharma screw up, Mom," he stated emphatically. "They create a new drug and tout it as the best invention since sliced bread. Everyone jumps on the bandwagon before long-term research is complete. Then someone abuses it. People panic, and it gets put in the dumpster. Now, finally, science is digging it out of the trash and figuring out a way to keep it from being abused so it can help people again."

"Money prompts that decision, I am sure," I interjected.

"Exactly! Without proper research and controls, it is easier to abuse."

I merely shrugged. "People will always abuse things, Luke. Even too much sunshine gets one burned."

"Whoa!" he exclaimed, getting into one of his "it's time to fight Mom because no one else is around" modes. "So let's just ban sunbathing? Let's restrict how many groceries fat people can buy? Let's ban everything we don't understand. How about guns? Want to go there?"

"I'm sorry, son. It was an insensitive remark," I said, genuinely remorseful. I had poked the bear but saw his point.

Luke nodded and continued with his original point. "The same thing happened with cocaine, you know. Freud used it as a numbing agent on most of his patients. He was even trying to cure his friend's morphine addiction with cocaine."[6]

"Freud? Really? How stupid!"

"Well, it works, Mom. It does cut the cravings."

"And how would you know?" I asked, suddenly fearful he would try anything to feel better.

Ignoring my question, he said, "In 1994, another study in a controlled environment tested Freud's work again."

"Seriously?" I asked in total disbelief.

He then pulled it up on PubMed: "Reduction of Opiate Withdrawal-Like Symptoms by Cocaine Abuse During Methadone and Buprenorphine Maintenance" by Stine and Kosten.[7]

"Here. Read." He shoved his computer on my lap.

"Well, then, why aren't more studies done?" I asked, pretty dumbfounded looking at the results.

"Because it's addictive and illegal," Luke retorted. "Plus, no one gives a shit, Mother! One percent of all the money spent on the opioid crisis goes to research and development. They think we are all junkies. I'm just trying to stay alive, Mom!" With that statement, he slammed the computer shut and left the room.

I went into the kitchen to process everything Luke shared with me. I was impressed with the legitimate new avenues scientists were exploring to treat SUD, like an innovative brain surgery doctors worked on at West Virginia University's Rockefeller Neuroscience Institute.[8] But the others seemed so unconventional. I was fighting the research because of the stigma attached. Meanwhile, Luke was digging in full force. *But why?* It soon became apparent Luke was getting desperate to recover. The old ways were failing, and he was looking for options—any option, as his brain was not healing. Dopamine depletion had set in, and we knew nothing about how to raise the levels.[9]

In the ensuing weeks, things did get better, but I could see Luke was still not himself. In the evenings, Luke insisted I watch odd foreign films with him about time travel, like *Dark* and *Beforeigners*, along with every episode of the new *Star Trek* series revolving around time travel and the gateway into the Vortex. I could not figure out why he was so engrossed in the topic of alternative existences and was fearfully beginning to wonder if Luke was afraid he might die.

One day I got brave enough to ask him if he was afraid he was dying and reminded him about his near-death experience after his accident.

"I only saw the portal, Mom; I didn't go through," was all he could muster.

*****

August was all about family. Luke and I were on the golf course almost daily, giving us time to dream and plan for his new life in North Carolina. Jim and Luke spent every Sunday morning watching Formula 1 races. Luke also spent a great deal of time with Worth and his family. We went to ball games, he took his nephew golfing and his niece on excursions, he went on cycling trips and to the pool, and he spent many evenings at Worth's house baking cookies and talking past midnight. Seeing him so happy again and connecting at such a deep level with his family was wonderful.

Luke also took off to Raleigh a few times to look at apartments—something close to the capital as he wanted to be close to the political

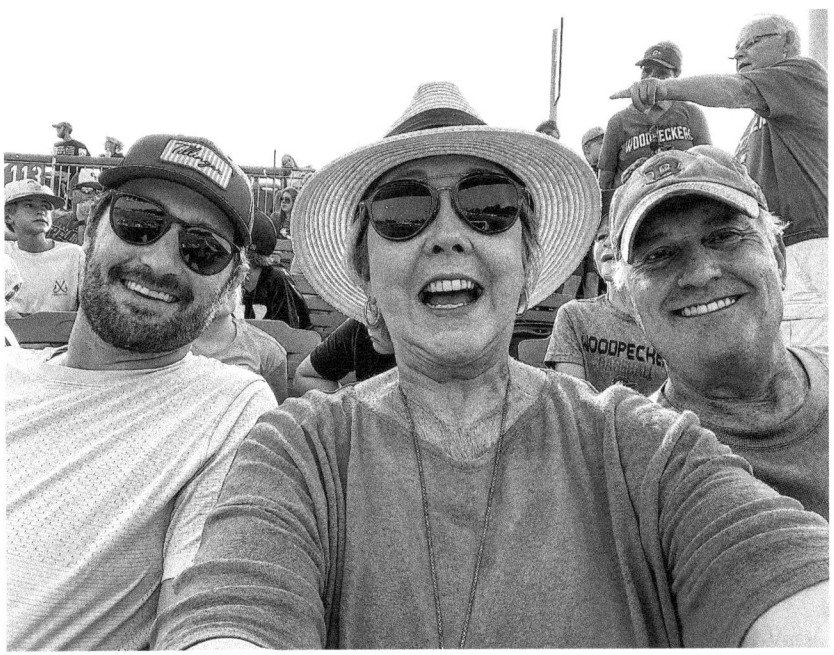

Family fun at a baseball game in July 2021: Luke, me and Jim.

action. He texted me pictures, asking my opinion and talking about all the good he could do, maybe even starting out as an aide to a congressman in his spare time.

He also dropped a bomb: he had been accepted to the Harvard Division of Continuing Education. He could take classes online toward a degree in political science. Again, I stood amazed that this kid who once was forced to get his GED had been accepted into two Ivy League non-traditional programs. He knew it was a challenging program and not the same as being a regular student at Harvard. Still, he was excited about the opportunity to take classes from some of the same professors and eventually get a degree that could get him into law school one day.

One day Luke bounded down the steps more excited than I had seen in months. "Hey, Mom, I am texting a beautiful woman I found on a dating site! I think she may be interested in me."

"Tell me about her," I asked with my usual nosiness.

"I think she's out of my league, but I reached out anyway. Today she texted back!"

"Young, petite blonde?" I joked.

"No. She is a tall brunette. She is also my age and owns her own swimsuit company. She is really smart. Her name is Lindsay, and she told me straight out she is looking to get married and wants to have children right away, so if that was not what I was looking for—end of conversation."

"Seriously? Seems like a woman who knows what she wants and does not want to waste time." I replied, a tad giddy.

"Exactly! I told her that's what I wanted too. I also told her my plans to finish my education and go into politics and my goals of making policy changes for the opioid crisis. I spelled out the timeframe because of my previous setbacks. She didn't care about the time—to her, it is all about being a team heading in the same direction."

A few days later, he bounced down the steps doing the Snoopy happy dance. "*Mom.* Lindsay and I are going out on a date."

"When?" I replied with the same excitement.

"When she gets back from a trip, in a week. I need a new suit!" he said with his "let's go shopping" grin. And so we did. But a few things still concerned me.

In early August, I put away clothes in Luke's room and found a large syringe in his drawer. I didn't panic but asked him for an answer. He was not shaken.

"Mom, you do see it's the size of a small turkey baster, don't you?" he said calmly.

"Oh ... yes," I responded, taking a good look at the size.

"One does not shoot up heroin with a turkey baster." We both laughed.

"Then what is it for?"

He pulled out a vial of testosterone, telling me his libido had been nonexistent for months.

"All my hormones are screwed up, and I'm just trying to get 'me' back," he said with a wink. Luke also told me he had started using kratom tea again.

"Be careful, Bug." Now I was really concerned.

"Mom, I had to stop the Suboxone because it was making me constipated, and I was only getting a few hours of sleep a night ... and my night terrors have returned. Damn side effects. The tea doesn't do that to me and also cuts the cravings."

"I know, but..." I said, trying to let him live his life but afraid of the tolerance effect as each time he used it, he would escalate back to narcotics.

Luke tried to calm my fears. "I have an appointment with my addictionologist a few days after I get back to LA. He will keep me balanced until my money comes in, and then I promise I will go into a good treatment center for as long as it takes."

"OK, Bug." I had to trust his judgment, but my fears were creeping back in at an alarming rate.

The evening Luke went back to his brother's to spend the night, but around 3 a.m., the dogs took off down our hallway barking. Our sentries were always waiting for his late-night entries.

"You home?" I texted Luke in a bit of a daze.

Ping. "Yes, sorry. I woke up in a panic and had this intense feeling that I had to go home to feel safe. Just felt like an impending feeling of doom. I'm OK now. Sorry about the dog alarm. See you in the morning." End of text.

His text sent a chill down my spine. He had another night terror. *What was happening to my son?*

*****

The next day Luke came down the steps to give me my morning hug. Usually, they were quickly followed with a peck on the forehead. Instead, he held me for the longest time without saying a word. I welcomed his embrace as it helped assuage my fears. The days could not come quickly enough for him to move back to North Carolina permanently.

Later that day, I caught him in the den staring out into the backyard. Quietly he said, "You are my greatest love, you know…"

"Oh, no, honey," I quickly replied. "I am your first love. One day I promise you will find your greatest love."

He was quiet for a moment before replying softly, "No … it's you."

*****

As the days passed, Luke got more excited about his date with Lindsay. They were texting multiple times a day, getting to know each better. In the afternoon of the 24th, Luke borrowed my car and took off to Raleigh. His suit had been tailored, and he could change clothes in the dressing room before his date. I honestly didn't expect to hear from him until he got home that night, but at 6:30, my phone pinged with a text.

"*Mom!* She's the most beautiful woman I have ever met. And fun!"

"Where is she now?" I texted back, wondering how he got away with texting me.

"In the bathroom—just had to tell you."

"Does she like you too?" I quickly shot back in my nosey fashion.

"Oh yes, she does. I'm definitely coming to Raleigh! Gotta go."

When he got home at 2 a.m., he was ecstatic. Naturally, the dogs alerted me to his arrival, and I went downstairs to greet him. I was so relieved to hear they had connected and a possible future together sounded promising.

We decided to play one last game of golf before he headed back to LA the following day. Though still tired from his late-night date, he was getting back his game. I was busy taking pictures and daydreaming about having him only an hour away. A storm hit midway through, sending us scrambling back to the clubhouse, careening over the cart paths and laughing as we got drenched. I was amazed that my son had turned into my best friend. Seeing hope return to his eyes was so good.

Chapter 10. The Perfect Storm

I usually dreaded his leaving but not this time. There would be much to do before he returned with his belonging in two weeks. My list was getting longer by the minute.

The following day we finished packing and headed to Raleigh early to choose between two apartments he had picked out. He told me Lindsay would help him decorate. They had been texting hourly. We then grabbed lunch before heading to the airport. I was barely able to contain my joy. My boy was coming home! OK, his new home, but he'd be close by. Visions of weekend stopovers, football games, and frequent family get-togethers raced through my head on the way to the airport.

Luke looked so handsome as he unloaded his bags, his new beige suit and white t-shirt showing off that beautiful, tanned face. Intentionally I didn't write him a special note for his suitcase this time as he was only going back to pack up his belongings and make final closure with his life in LA. My little boy had grown into the most wonderful, competent man amidst chaos, tragedy, and disease. I was so proud.

Instead of our usual long, drawn-out hugs, kisses, and goodbyes, Luke simply turned to me quickly, putting both hands on my shoulders, and said, "This is not goodbye, Momma. I will see you in two weeks. I love you." With a quick kiss and hug, he was gone.

I got in the car, smiling, and looked at my watch. 3:20 p.m. Phew. His flight was at 5:00. For once, he was on time. He texted me as usual upon his arrival. As always, I couldn't sleep until I heard he was home safe.

The following day, however, Luke called me in a full-on panic attack. He could not hear, was dizzy, and could not stand without falling over. We ported over to texting because he could not hear my replies. Something was defiantly amiss. I had not heard him this freaked out since the accident that almost took his life. I was afraid. But what could I do? He was grown. I was 3,000 miles away. I explained to him that what he was experiencing was commonly called "airplane ear"—blocked Eustachian tubes. I tried to reassure him that he would be all right in a few hours. His anxiety was too intense to heed my advice—he needed help at this moment and left to find it. I prayed.

Luke did check in later in the day, texting that he was OK, that he had just been terrified that he'd never be able to listen to music again. I didn't ask questions when he later texted me the clinic line was three hours long. He told me not to worry, reminding me that his addictionologist appointment was in a few days.

But I was still scared. Something didn't feel right. I knew so many things in Luke's brain were starting to fail. I suspected he found a pharmaceutical intervention that brought his anxiety down. I prayed it was from a safe source.

Jim and I went to bed early that Friday night. In the early morning hours, around 3, the dogs woke us with a start and bolted down the hallway barking loudly as they always did when Luke came home late. "How odd," Jim mumbled as they came back, their tails wagging.

Jim asked, "Luke's in LA, right?" I whispered, "Yes."

Since I was now awake, I decided to check and see if Luke had replied to my texts or if there was any activity on our joint bank account—Luke was always ordering Uber Eats or getting something from the corner store.

Nothing.

Crawling back into bed, I had the most horrific feeling of terror-filled anxiety come over me. Its weight was crushing and frightening enough to make me think about whether I had anything in the medicine cabinet to calm it down. *Perhaps Luke left a Klonopin—or three?* Then I heard Luke's voice. Not in my ears or in my head, but directly through my heart: "Momma, I just had to show you the feelings I have been forced to live with for so long so you'd understand. I love you…" And then the feeling subsided.

Sleep never came that night. I went to my fallback feeling: numb. All day I tried texting and checking accounts. Still nothing. I was frozen. Another night came and went without sleep.

I feared the worst early Sunday morning and called the police for a welfare check. I fully expected them to call back and tell me he had overdosed but was still alive. He had such a high tolerance and always pulled through. I used to call him Teflon.

The moment I heard the policeman draw a breath, I knew what he would say. There was a slow and deliberate inhale. Time stood still as he dreaded words left his lips: "I'm sorry, ma'am. Phone calls like this are never easy. There is not a kind way to say this … your son is deceased."

Chapter 11

Dying for Change

"Memories saturate my heart and the story of you spills from my eyes."—Grace Andren

Shock, disbelief, and pain beyond comprehension took turns punching me in the stomach as I slowly fell to my knees, gasping for breath. Not my son. My only child. My baby! Dearest God, *no!*

Surely this was a waking nightmare. It couldn't be true. My mind was racing through the memories trying to make sense of the senseless. We had just spent the past two and a half months together, having the time of our lives. Luke was healing, golfing, cooking, being the fun brother, wise uncle, and loving, adoring son. He had made plans to leave California and move back to North Carolina to be closer to us all. He had found a classy new girlfriend. I bought him new custom golf clubs, two designer suits, and a first-class ticket back to LA. He was so excited to come home. He had so much to live for, and suddenly, he was gone.

Time stood still. Shock set in. Blessed, numbing shock. In a daze, I called his brothers and Jenni, breaking the news as I paced around the kitchen island. An hour later, the police investigator called. He filled us in on the details calmly, asking if Luke had a history of drug use.

"Yes, it was the price we paid for his life after his accident," I mumbled weakly.

"OK. That explains the scars all over his body. We were wondering," he responded in an acknowledging tone.

"I know. Not your typical drug addict, right?" I knew all too well the stigma attached to an overdose victim.

"Does not look that way, ma'am. I am so sorry for your loss."

Cautiously I asked, "When did he pass? Can you tell? Was it last night?"

"I can't be sure, Susan, but after doing these investigations for more than 25 years, I would estimate he has been gone about 32 hours. He did not appear to have suffered, but it has all the earmarks of an accidental overdose. Fentanyl poisoning, most likely. The coroner's report will give you the details in a few days. Again, I am sorry for your loss," he answered respectfully.

Again, my knees gave out as I thanked the detective and ended the call. My precious boy had been dead on his bathroom floor alone all that time? The thought was too much to bear. I ran outside screaming, doubled over, trying to keep from retching up my soul. Jim tried to calm me, but I was inconsolable. It then hit me as I counted back the hours; Luke passed away late Friday, around midnight Pacific time—3 a.m. our time. It was the exact time the dogs barked, and I felt his presence trying to explain the unexplainable. The world as I knew it forever faded away before my eyes.

The next day my friend Susan Lee called to express her condolences. I had not been answering the phone, but I took the call when I saw who it was. Susan was an intuitive soul and had unique gifts since experiencing an NDE as a child. I, too, had a sense of the unexplained since Luke shared his experience after his accident.

After the usual condolences, she said timidly, "I just had to call you and tell you about a vivid dream I had the other night. I've been frightened to tell you as I don't want you to think I am crazy. It was so real! I swear I am not making this up, but the urge to share this with you won't go away."

"It's OK. I'm beyond crazy with grief now. Tell me about the dream," I numbly replied.

She went on in trepidation, "I had a vision and saw Luke fall to the floor in his bathroom. Then I saw his grandmother was there. She reached down into him and lifted his spirit up in her arms. There were other golden orbs there, too, which led him upwards. He was never alone, Susan. I swear I am not making this up to make you feel better." Her voice trailed off.

A sudden peace surrounded me as chills ran down my arms. "Thank you, Susan," I replied with a newfound calm. "I don't think you are crazy. Luke's grandmother always told him she was his angel and would never leave him. She loved him so much. Thank you for telling me. Truly," I said, ending the call.

Chapter 11. Dying for Change

I chose to accept her words as truth. My terror had abated, allowing me to take in the unthinkable and move on, making plans to bring my son home.

I don't remember much from the following days. Thank heavens I had help. Jenni dropped everything and drove 16 hours through the night to be by my side. Jim made the arrangements with a funeral home in LA. It was backed up and would need at least 10 days to cremate his body and ship his ashes home. At least that gave me time to write Luke's obituary and plan his memorial service. My numbness was deployed for me to move forward. Thank God it was available or I would not have been able to keep my sanity.

We had to deal with unpleasant details. The coroner's report revealed that Luke had indeed succumbed to fentanyl poisoning. Luke's friends cleaned his apartment and express-shipped me his personal belongings. I received them and saw Luke's iPhone was locked but his iWatch was not. Desperate to know the details of his final hours, I pulled up his messages. There in front of me was the answer. During his panic attack, he contacted an old friend. The text detailed his plea for relief from his anxiety and cravings. She wrote back, arranging a meeting. Instantly I called the police with the information, telling them I had found my son's murderer.

The cold reply cut through me like a knife. "Los Angeles does not prosecute drug dealers of this nature. I am sorry for your loss." Click.

Life was surreal. The days dragged on as I sat on the front porch waiting for a swatch of Luke's hair from the kindly mortician.

The day before Luke's wake, Jim and I were waiting for his remains to arrive at a park close to the funeral home. In a haze, my mind returned to the last time I saw my son at the airport. His words echoed through my mind: *"I'm not saying goodbye, Momma. I'll be back in two weeks. I love you!"*

The ping from Jim's phone brought me back into the present moment. It was the text telling us Luke's ashes had arrived. I looked at my watch as I gathered my belongings: 3:20. A chill went through me as a cardinal was in my path to the car. It was exactly two weeks to the day, hour, and minute Luke told me he'd be back home. Grace took over. God knew. Luke was indeed home. No more pain. No more anxiety or depression. No screws in his back, no rods. No more surgeries. No more drugs. My baby was at peace.

*****

Some people were stunned when I shared in Luke's obituary that along with all his incredible accomplishments, he had SUD and died of an unsuccessful attempt at self-medication. *Why?* At his wake, eyes avoided mine as people expressed their condolences. *Why?* After his service, many people didn't know what to say. *Why? Why were they so uncomfortable?* I was not ashamed of my son. Would they have reacted the same way if Luke had died of cancer? Stigma told them my son got weak and wanted to get high. Stigma told them I must be terribly ashamed of my child. Stigma withheld their love and comfort hostage.

How my son died did not define his life. Luke was not a morally deficient drug addict, as the world would have you believe of people that suffer from SUD. Luke was a successful businessman and college student. He was brilliant, funny, spiritual, kind, and thoughtful. Luke was my hero and fought a noble fight. He outmaneuvered death, taking the devil on time and time again with determination and grace. I was very proud of how my son lived his short life and not ashamed he died of a disease. *Why were they?*

The scientific truth is that my son was sick. He had a chronic genetic disease called substance use disorder. His brain was predisposed to it and, over time, his brain had been damaged by narcotics and the other toxic drugs used to get him off the original ones. He did not fail himself or me. The medical community failed him. Insurance failed him. Public policy failed him.

People with SUD are not their disease. They are not all "junkies." They are doctors, lawyers, bus drivers, teachers, judges, nurses, soldiers, students, factory workers, cooks, cleaners, grandmothers, mothers, fathers, uncles, aunts, and children. Those poor souls we see on the street curbs or in jail are the people who have no support systems, no money, no insurance, no treatment, and no hope. Even those who begin using drugs to get high or avoid emotional pain are blindly unaware of the brain-altering addictive properties of narcotics. No one intentionally chooses to become dependent on drugs.

Substance use disorder is a neglected disease due to stigma

surrounding drug use, and its treatment is still caught up in the dark ages. My son was not to blame for his disease. Science has proven there are neurobiological genetic and social precursors that set specific individuals up for SUD.[1] These discoveries take the onus off the individual, allowing him the chance to have proper care and respect. Yet most of this information lies dormant in scientific journals that are unobtainable and unreadable to laypersons and policymakers. *Why?*

Although clinical research has advanced, the pharmaceutical companies, the medical community, public policy, and outdated and inaccurate cultural beliefs are still decades behind in their understanding of SUD. Public policy restricts care as it still blames individuals for their disease. *Why?*

There are too many unanswered *whys* that demand answers.

Why is there so little money allocated for research for a cure? *Why* are there no safe avenues for emergency medications or treatment centers for SUD patients? *Why* can any physician, physician assistant, or nurse practitioner prescribe narcotics but can't prescribe Suboxone without specialized training? *Why* don't surgeons and medical personnel know to treat people with SUD with safe protocols that help avoid relapse? *Why* doesn't every ED have Suboxone or Methadone available to treat those with SUD? *Why* is MOUD not available to all who request it? *Why* don't insurance companies pay for a complete treatment knowing it takes an average of 14–16 months of sobriety for an addict's brain to balance neurotransmitter levels with a neuro-typical brain? *Why* aren't sobriety houses covered by insurance when they have been proven to provide optimal time for brain recovery? *Why* do insurance companies only allow only one treatment per year? *Why* does the AA community insist those who are dual diagnosis and on medication to balance their brain chemistry are not really sober and/or working the program? *Why* don't people know that SUD is not a moral deficiency that cannot be solved by only going to AA/NA meetings?

The blaming needs to stop. We need to do better. The paradigm needs to change. Insurance benefits need to change. Public awareness needs to change. Public policy needs to change. The medical community must be trained to deal with this disease without prejudice.

My son lived his life hoping to create policy changes for a misunderstood and undertreated disease. He suffered unmercifully at the

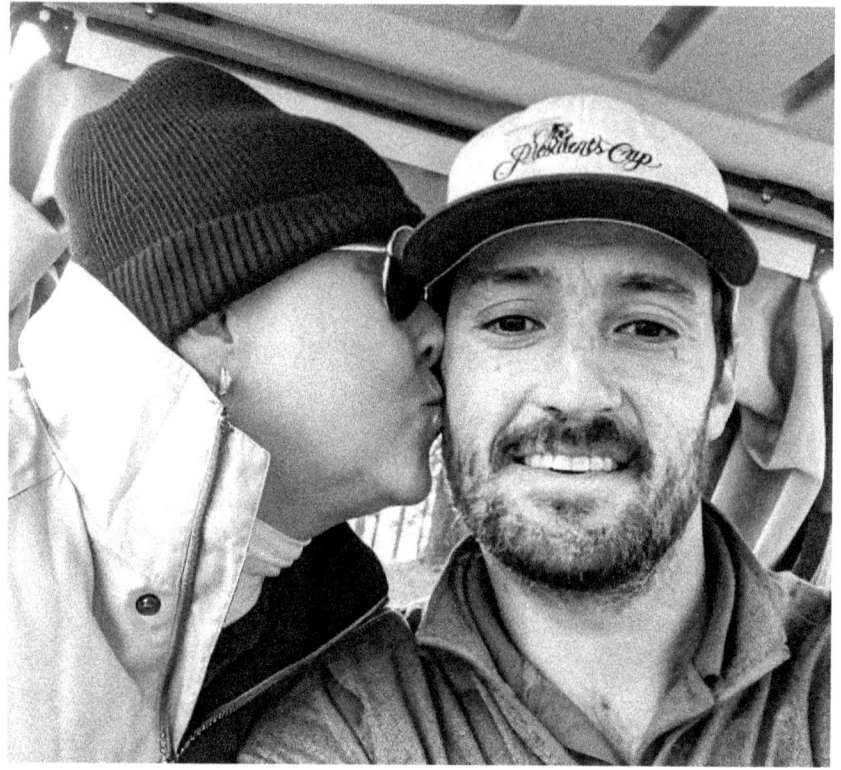

Goodbye sweetheart—I'll see you on the other side.

hands of the medical establishment, who are bound by an oath to do no harm. He struggled to make the world a better place by creating a natural product with proven efficacy to help anxiety tied up in red tape and ignorance. He panicked because his system could not function properly anymore, and he felt he had no other option but to go to the street during a mental health crisis.

My son died trying to make a change. He can do no more. Now it's up to us.

Goodbye, sweetheart. I'll see you on the other side. Until then, I will fight for you and all the other people who have lost loved ones to substance use disorder. Your life was not in vain. I love you *forever and always*. Momma.

Robert Luke Paschal
1991–2021

Afterword

BY ARUN GUPTA, M.D.

Addiction Provider and Author of:
The Preventable Epidemic: A Frontline Doctor's Experience and Recommendations to Resolve America's Opioid Crisis

The opioid crisis is growing at an exponential rate. In 1999, 4,000 people died of a narcotic overdose. Today it has become an epidemic claiming over more than one million people at the rate of 300 people per day. That is a 25,000 percent increase in deaths from unintentional overdoses. The current war on drugs strategy is obviously unsuccessful. Yet, as a nation, we focus on the substances decimating our young population and ignore the bio-neurological disease at the core of substance use disorder (SUD). Simply going after the drug cartels will not stop the carnage.

As a medical physician treating patients with substance and opioid use disorder for more than 17 years, I have seen firsthand the devastation and heartbreak caused to those afflicted and their families.

One reason for the crisis is the lack of addiction providers. Recent reports from the American Society of Addiction Medicine (ASAM) indicate that 41 million people in America are at risk of dying from substance use disorder, with only 2.4 million in treatment. The remaining 39 million have no access to care. This highlights a severe lack of addiction providers, regulatory blunders, misclassification of prescribed remedies, failed policies, and the public's lack of demand for necessary and effective changes due to stigma.

The government's response to the crisis has failed to address the issue effectively. Social organizations and big employers have not stepped up to the plate despite the availability of an effective medicine, Suboxone, which has been approved since September 2002. Medications for opioid use disorder are the gold standards for treatment and essential for dual diagnosis patients. Yet using MOUD has been shunned by insurance companies and policymakers as they still base their recommendations on the original 1935 dictates that addiction is a moral failing and can only be cured through the 12 Step program.

Suboxone, a Class 3 drug, was approved in 2002 for doctors to prescribe in in-office settings for narcotic addiction. However, a diversion control plan was started in 2005, reinforcing the treatment arm's criminalization. This worsened when Ricketts/Indivior was sued for $2 billion as Suboxone was diverted on the street. While there have been some efforts to address the opioid crisis, they have been inadequate. Of the 331.9 million people in the United States, approximately 950,000 (0.29 percent) are physicians. The total number of addiction practitioners with the necessary credentials to treat SUD is 138,000. The passage of DATA 2000 allowed doctors to be labeled as addiction providers. Yet today, fewer than 7,000 provide care to the 2.4 million afflicted by SUD.

The lack of access to care coupled with deadlier street drugs has been the main reason for escalating overdose deaths, now overtaken by street fentanyl. The failure to effectively improve access to care has resulted in 39 million people at risk of having no access to prescriptions written by a doctor for Suboxone/Buprenorphine. The lack of access and not abuse is the leading cause of diversion.

Although Naloxone has helped to reduce overdose deaths, it is no longer enough to reverse the effects of fentanyl and carfentanyl. The standard Narcan is ineffective; even multiple dosages cannot save lives. The tragic reality is that even middle school students are dying from accidental fentanyl poisoning.

The failure to mandate educational requirements for addiction medicine in American medical schools is another reason the opioid crisis continues to grow. The National College of Academic Addiction Medicine claims that only 96 fellowships are accredited by the Accreditation Council for Graduate Medical Education. Compare that to the American Medical Association's 5,110 specialty programs and 11,767 fellowship positions for 2020–2021.

While some regulations have been enforced to curb the pills and pill mills, they have resulted in more than 1,000 providers being apprehended for overprescribing these restricted medication classes. This has further discouraged other providers from learning and practicing addiction medicine. Ironically, doctors are not permitted to prescribe Methadone, a Class 2 drug stronger than Suboxone, a Class 3 drug, for treating addiction but can prescribe other Class 2 drugs that are equally addictive and abusive. The availability of Methadone is limited to federal programs called OTPs, which are not easily accessible to those in rural areas where treatment is needed the most.

If the Accreditation Council for Graduate Medical Education (ACGME) had started teaching addiction medicine in American medical schools in the year 2000, there would have been 500,000 new doctors fully trained to tackle this crisis. ACGME is still not mandating educational requirements to teach and learn addiction in medical schools universally, even until 2022.

More than 100,000 people will lose their lives yearly unless we make substantial policy changes. Failure to act will result in millions more people dying of fentanyl poisoning and/or unintentional overdose by 2030.

According to the World Health Organization, addiction to illicit drugs is the most stigmatizing condition. Like other stigmatized diseases of the past, mental disorders, AIDS, venereal diseases, leprosy, and certain skin diseases, our mindset must change about SUD to turn around the opioid epidemic. It is time to come out of the dark ages and follow science.

First, we must acknowledge that SUD is a genetic and metabolic disease. Diseases are treated by making treatment options available to everyone afflicted and providing nondiscriminatory support and preventative measures.

To provide adequate care, medical schools must reconfigure their curriculum to include a frank discussion of how addiction can be prevented, how to spot it, and how to direct patients to treatment. Hospitals and medical doctors would benefit by forming better alliances with behavioral health centers. Every medical professional in America needs mandatory education on addiction, empathy, proper vocabulary, and humanity. We can only start to reduce stigma; otherwise, it is just another talking point.

Addiction treatment must fully integrate into mainstream healthcare by providing sustainable funding through personal and private insurance coverage. Sobriety houses that use MOUD should be subsidized.

Politicians must be prohibited from accepting donations from Big Pharma. The advertising of pharmaceuticals on television also needs to be examined.

Grants must become available for research for a cure, and a more significant part of the funding for fighting the war on drugs should go to research.

The government should provide free MOUD—Suboxone and Narcan—to anyone who needs it.

Lastly, we must encourage the public health community to work with law enforcement to move away from incarceration toward treatment-centered programs. Local police stations now get rewarded for drug busts. They must be rewarded for using Suboxone and treatment counselors to save lives.

Together we can make a change. More than one million people have died. We must act before you or a family member becomes one of those million.

Acknowledgments

First, I would like to thank Jacob Taylor. As Luke's best friend, you immediately turned your pain into action, demanding his story be told to save others. Your constant encouragement allowed me to put his story into book form. Thank you for your efforts, and Tom Foran and Justin Ross for turning it into a screenplay. Truly, Luke's story will now see the light of day because of your love and support.

A special thank you to my good friend and first editor, Christine Arvidson. Serendipity brought us together as college roommates. Fate brought us back together after 40 years. You took the ramblings of a grieving mother and showed me how to turn them into a book, not to mention tenderly walking me through my grammatical blunders and introducing me to McFarland. Your friendship is invaluable.

Chas Allen, thank you from the bottom of my heart for compiling an excellent book proposal and editing three of the most critical chapters in the book. Your kindness throughout the entire process will forever be appreciated.

Special thanks to Susan Kilby, managing editor, and the entire team at McFarland, for believing in me and Luke's story that will hopefully save lives.

Dr. Rebecca Estes is a beloved friend, a medical advisor, and the light down my path that kept me moving forward throughout these past 20 years. The angels can only match your love and devotion to Luke and me. I can't thank you enough, and I'm so grateful God placed you in my life. And thank you for introducing me to the wise Tom Thomson of the Awakened Heart community—another bright light down my path.

I first heard addiction specialist Dr. Arun Gupta on Angela

Kennecke's podcast *Grieving Out Loud*. Dr. Gupta's vast knowledge of the topic impressed me, so I reached out for his support as an endorser for this book. He was gracious enough to do so and offered to step in as a medical adviser. He was true to his word and has walked every step of this process with me. Although not touched personally by this opioid crisis, he has dedicated his life to saving the lives of people afflicted with SUD (substance use disorder). Thank you, Arun, for your kindness and your expertise. The world is a better place because of you.

I also sincerely thank Dr. Thomas Buchheit, director of Duke Regenerative Pain Therapies Program. Thank you for being more than an experienced physician managing Luke's pain. You were Luke's only physician in this journey who showed love, compassion, expert knowledge of SUD, and genuine caring for him, our whole family, and our struggles. Also, I want to give you a special thanks for all the research you are doing to create alternative pain management treatments without using opioids. You are improving pain management care, and we thank you.

A heartfelt thanks to my husband, my rock, and the love of my life, James Herrick. You patiently kept fires burning while I incessantly wrote. At night you held me as I cried. You were a friend and mentor to my son and made our family whole. I love you, sweetheart.

Jenni Bradfield, if I had a daughter, it would be you. As your aunt, I was there to love and nurture you as a child. As an adult, you returned the favor by constantly showing up for me in times of crisis. Never was there a time I called that you did not drop everything and drive cross country to help me without hesitation. I love and thank you more than you know.

A special thank you to Luke's first love, Yarrow Courney. You selflessly interrupted your life to care for my son and mother when I could not. Your deep friendship with Luke and my entire family remained even after your romantic relationship ended. I am grateful to call you family and to thank you for still gracing my life with your beautiful presence. As Jim says, you are our bonus daughter.

A profound, heartfelt thanks to my stepson Worth Paschal and his wife, Alecia. Though there was 20 years difference between you and Luke, you were always his faithful and caring full brother. Through all the difficult times, your steadfastness, intellect, and deep love of family were an anchor we could always count on. I thank you, a district attorney, for pushing forward in the criminal court system by establishing drug courts now aimed toward treatment over incarceration. You are a brave, caring man.

Thank you for your years of love and support, Marcia Sheppard Johnson. Together we walked, hand in hand, watching our children suffer, helpless to find relief or a cure. We lost our children within four months of each other and held each other up. I know Luke and Kelly are together guiding us forward. Until we hold them again, I love you.

To the Rev. John Hage, thank you for the beautiful eulogy you gave my son. Your words showed what unbiased love looks like and how all those who suffer need love without judgment. Your messages of compassion inspired us all. And a loving thanks to those special people at Brownson Memorial Presbyterian Church who loved and devotedly supported Luke, especially Caryl Peterson, Deryle Carr, Reggie Reid, Jeanette Wilson, Katherine Ewing, Cynthia Strickland, Janie Gould, Terry Brown, Lu Sims, Katherine Marsh, ZoeAnn and David Cagle, Missy and Henry Brown, Nancy and Bob Weant, and the late Michael Howe.

Thanks also to my UNC and Fayetteville State University and Shaklee colleagues who kept my ball rolling when I could not: Phoebe Hall, Dave Griffee, Todd Frobish, Torin Wright, Moyra Gorski, Pam Carey, Jennifer Glacken, Roger Barnett, Marjorie Fine, Dr. Bruce Daggy, Dr. Jamie McManus, and Wanda Hart.

Lastly, to all the angels on earth who have lost children and geared their pain toward fighting the opioid crisis. My heartfelt thanks to Angela Kennecke for founding Emily's Hope; Pam Sugarman Moules for her unremitting efforts through For Jonathan's Sake—Steps4Hope Foundation; Brenda Richards Schivito, founder of Angels Against Addiction; and "The Pharmacist" Daniel Schneider for his relentless fight to get MAT (medication-assisted treatment) free of charge to everyone who needs it. And to all parents who have lost a child who now fight the war on drugs so no one else will ever have to die needlessly, let us continue to make the world a better place in honor and in memory of our children.

Chapter Notes

Chapter 1

1. "The *DSM* is the *Diagnostic and Statistical Manual of Mental Disorders* in psychology and psychiatry. This is a manual that is used as a standard across the profession for diagnosing and treating mental disorders. Within the *DSM*'s pages are diagnostic codes used for billing purposes and data collection by mental health providers across the country. Each disorder listed in the manual features a specific set of diagnostic criteria that must be adhered to when diagnosing a mental disorder. Symptoms and the duration of symptoms must be present in the patient before a clinician can reach a true diagnosis." Reference.com, last updated April 2, 2020.

2. "Controversy Over DSM-5: New Mental Health Guide," *Nursing Times*, August 24, 2013. https://www.nursingtimes.net/news/behind-the-headlines/controversy-over-dsm-5-new-mental-health-guide-24-08-2013/.

3. For a description of night terrors, see Ngoc L. Van Horn and Megan Street, "Night Terrors," *StatPearls*, January 2023, last updated May 29, 2023. PMID: 29630274. https://pubmed.ncbi.nlm.nih.gov/29630274/.

4. Mostafa Hemamy, Naseh Pahlavani, Alireza Amanollahi, Sheikh Mohammed Shriful Islam, Jenna McVicar, Gholamreza Askari, and Mahsa Malekahmadi, "The Effect of Vitamin D and Magnesium Supplementation on the Mental Health Status of Attention-Deficit Hyperactive Children: A Randomized Controlled Trial," *BMC Pediatrics* 21, no. 1 (April 17, 2021): 178. doi: 10.1186/s12887-021-02631-1.

5. "Attention deficit hyperactivity disorder (ADHD) is the most common comorbid condition in patients with Tourette syndrome (TS). The co-occurrence of ADHD and TS is often associated with a higher social and psychopathological impairment. Comorbidity between Tourette's and ADHD appears to have a complex and partially known pathogenesis in which genetic, environmental, and neurobiological factors can be implicated." Nadia El-Malhany, Mariangela Gulisano, Renata Rizzo, and Paolo Curatolo, "Tourette Syndrome and Comorbid ADHD: Causes and Consequences," *European Journal of Pediatrics* 174, no. 3 (March 2015): 279–288. doi: 10.1007/s00431-014-2417-0. PMID: 25224657.

6. "Magnesium Shown to Calm Hyperactivity in Children," E.I.N. Newswires, September 30, 2022. https://www.einnews.com/pr_news/592794090/magnesium-shown-to-calm-hyperactivity-in-children. Mohammad Effatpanah, Mahdi Rezaei, Hosein Effatpanah, Zeynab Effatpanah, Hamed Kord Varkaneh, Seyed Mohammad Mousavi, Somaye Fatahi, Giulia Rinaldi, and Rezvan Hashemi, "Magnesium Status and Attention Deficit Hyperactivity Disorder (ADHD): A Meta-Analysis," *Psychiatry Research* 274 (April 2019): 228–234. https://www.sciencedirect.com/science/article/abs/pii/S0165178118318456.

7. "Misuse of prescription stimulants can lead to a substance use disorder (SUD), which takes the form of addiction in severe cases. Long-term use of stimulants, even as prescribed by a doctor, can cause a person to develop a tolerance, which

means that he or she needs higher and/or more frequent doses of the drug to get the desired effects. SUD develops when continued use of the drug causes issues, such as health problems and failure to meet responsibilities at work, school, or home. Concerns about use should be discussed with a healthcare provider." National Institute on Drug Abuse, "Prescription Stimulants DrugFacts," National Institutes of Health, U.S. Department of Health & Human Services, June 2018. https://nida.nih.gov/publications/drugfacts/prescription-stimulants. Also see "Adderall Neurotoxicity from Misuse," Oxford Treatment Center. https://oxfordtreatment.com/prescription-drug-abuse/adderall/neurotoxicity/, updated May 23, 2023.

8. Chantelle Pattemore, "How Do Adderall and Meth (Methamphetamine) Differ?" Healthline, January 20, 2023, medically reviewed by Philip Ngo, PharmD. https://www.healthline.com/health/adhd/how-do-adderall-and-meth-methamphetamine.

Chapter 2

1. For a list of the precursors to addiction, see Emma J. Rose, Giorgia Picci and Diana H. Fishbien, "Neurocognitive Precursors of Substance Misuse Corresponding to Risk, Resistance, and Resilience Pathways: Implications for Prevention Science," *Frontiers in Society* 10 (June 14, 2019). https://www.frontiersin.org/articles/10.3389/fpsyt.2019.00399/full.

2. Carlie Porterfield, "These Museums Still Have the Sackler Name Up Despite Opioid Crisis Controversy," *Forbes*, May 29, 2018. https://www.forbes.com/sites/carlieporterfield/2022/02/07/these-museums-still-have-the-sackler-name-up-despite-opioid-crisis-controversy/?sh=405ae6b857d5.

3. Substance Abuse and Mental Health Service Administration (SAMHSA), "Buprenorphine," U.S. Department of Health & Human Services. https://www.samhsa.gov/medications-substance-use-disorders/medications-counseling-related-conditions/buprenorphine, last updated July 18, 2023.

4. Joseph Pergolizzi, Jo Ann K. LeQuang, and Frank Breve, "The End of the X-Waiver: Not a Moment Too Soon!" *Cureus* 13, no. 5 (May 19, 2021): e15123. doi: 10.7759/cureus.15123. PMID: 34159025; PMCID: PMC8212919. https://pubmed.ncbi.nlm.nih.gov/34159025/.

5. Ben A. Rich, "Physicians' Legal Duty to Relieve Suffering," *The Western Journal of Medicine* 175, no. 3 (September 2001): 151–152. doi: 10.1136/ewjm.175.3.151. PMID: 11527832; PMCID: PMC1071521.

6. Alfred Clavel, Jr., M.D., "5 Ways Opioids and Their Negative Side Effects Make Your Pain Worse," Health Partners, accessed January 1, 2023. https://www.healthpartners.com/blog/why-opioids-make-pain-worse/.

Chapter 3

1. "A person may develop tolerance to a drug when the drug is used repeatedly. For instance, when morphine or alcohol is used for a long time, larger and larger doses must be taken to produce the same effect. Usually, tolerance develops because metabolism of the drug speeds up (often because the liver enzymes involved in metabolizing drugs become more active) and because the number of sites (cell receptors) that the drug attaches to or the strength of the bond (affinity) between the receptor and drug decreases)." Shalini S. Lynch, PharmD, "Tolerance and Resistance to Drugs," *Merck Manual Online*. https://www.merckmanuals.com/home/drugs/factors-affecting-response-to-drugs/tolerance-and-resistance-to-drugs, full review/revision July 2022, modified September 2022.

2. Jan Hoffman, "Most Doctors Are Ill-Equipped to Deal with the Opioid Epidemic. Few Medical Schools Teach Addiction," *New York Times*, September 10, 2018. https://www.nytimes.com/2018/09/10/health/addiction-medical-schools-treatment.html. This article details the lack of medical training in America today. It states, "Comprehensive addiction training is rare in American medical education. A report by the National Center on Addiction and Substance Abuse at Columbia University called out 'the failure of the medical profession at every level— in medical school, residency training,

continuing education and in practice' to adequately address addiction.'"

3. Louis Lasagna, "The Hippocratic Oath: Modern Version," *Nova*, January 1, 1964. https://www.pbs.org/wgbh/nova/doctors/oath_modern.html.

4. Shraddha Chakradhar and Casey Ross, "The History of OxyContin, Told Through Unsealed Purdue Documents," STAT, December 3, 2019. https://www.statnews.com/2019/12/03/oxycontin-history-told-through-purdue-pharma-documents/.

5. National Institute on Drug Abuse, "Drug Overdose Death Rates," National Institutes of Health, U.S. Department of Health & Human Services, February 9, 2019. https://nida.nih.gov/research-topics/trends-statistics/overdose-death-rates.

6. "Every day, approximately 220 Americans die after overdosing on opioids. Combining opioids and benzodiazepines can increase risk of overdose because both types of drugs can cause sedation and suppress breathing—the cause of overdose fatality—in addition to impairing cognitive functions. Research shows that people who use opioids and benzodiazepines concurrently are at higher risk of visiting the emergency department, being admitted to a hospital for a drug-related emergency, and dying of drug overdose." National Institute on Drug Abuse, "Co-Prescribing Opioids and Benzodiazepines," National Institutes of Health, U.S. Department of Health & Human Services, November 27, 2022. https://nida.nih.gov/research-topics/opioids/benzodiazepines-opioids.

7. Fred Upton, "Drug Overdose Death Rates. PRESCRIPTION DRUG DIVERSION: COMBATING THE SCOURGE," Subcommittee on Commerce, Manufacturing, and Trade, U.S. House of Representatives, March 1, 2012. energycommerce.house.gov.

8. "Failure to monitor and treat the symptoms of opiate withdrawal can (and does) result in death. Contrary to popular wisdom, death from acute opiate withdrawal is uncommon but not unprecedented. Withdrawal symptoms may include nausea, fever, sweating, vomiting, diarrhea, and hypertension. If left untreated, persistent vomiting and diarrhea can result in heart failure caused by hypernatraemia (elevated blood sodium levels) as well as severe dehydration." Katie Zuber, Patricia Stratch, and Elizabeth Pérez-Chiqués, "Five Myths of the Opioid Crisis," Rockefeller Institute of Government, February 7, 2019. https://rockinst.org/blog/five-myths-of-the-opioid-crisis/.

9. "With continued use, opioids change the chemistry. When a person takes a drug such as morphine or illicit heroin, the drug enters the central nervous system in the brain and binds to receptors known as 'opioid receptors' or 'mu receptors.' These receptors are located in areas of the brain known as the 'reward pathway' (cerebral cortex, nucleus accumbens, etc.) and 'pain pathway' (brainstem, spinal cord, thalamus, etc.). When binding to the pain pathway, opioids provide pain relief; however, when binding to the reward pathway, opioids cause euphoria and release a key neurotransmitter known as dopamine. Dopamine signals the body's neurons (brain or nerve cells) to create a pleasurable feeling or 'high.' The brain is naturally circuited to repeat processes that trigger the reward pathway. Therefore, this may lead to repeated use of the opioid in order to trigger the reward pathway again. However, the next time the opioid is taken will never be the same as the first." "Opioids and the Brain," PursueCare, April 10, 2019. https://www.pursuecare.com/opioids-and-the-brain/. Orna Levran, Vadim Yuferov, and Mary Jeanne Kreek, "The Genetics of the Opioid System and Specific Drug Addictions," *Human Genetics* 131, no. 6 (June 2012): 823–842. doi: 10.1007/s00439-012-1172-4. PMID: 22547174; PMCID: PMC3721349.

10. "The Opioid Pendulum: When Feeling Good Starts to Feel Bad": "It is the surge of withdrawal from opioids that makes the drugs so inescapable. Opioid addiction becomes entrenched after a person's neurons adapt to the drugs. The GABAergic neurons and other nerves in the brain still want to send messages, so they begin to adjust. They produce three to four times more cyclic AMP, a compound that primes the neuron to fire electric pulses, said Thomas Kosten, director of the division of alcohol and addiction psychiatry at the Baylor College of Medicine. That means even when you

take away the opioids, Kosten says, 'the neurons fire extensively.' The pendulum swings back. Now, rather than causing constipation and slowing respiration, the brain stem triggers diarrhea and elevates blood pressure. Instead of triggering happiness, the nucleus accumbens and amygdala reinforce feelings of dysphoria and anxiety. All of this negativity feeds into the prefrontal cortex, further pushing a desire for opioids. While other drugs like cocaine and alcohol can also feed addiction through the brain's pleasure circuits, it is the surge of withdrawal from opioids that makes the drugs so inescapable." Nsikan Akpan and Julia Griffin, "How a Brain Gets Hooked on Opioids," *PBS News Hour*, October 9, 2017. https://www.pbs.org/newshour/science/brain-gets-hooked-opioids.

11. "Posttraumatic stress disorder (PTSD) is a psychiatric disorder that may occur in people who have experienced or witnessed a traumatic event, series of events, or set of circumstances. An individual may experience this as emotionally or physically harmful or life-threatening, affecting mental, physical, social, and/or spiritual well-being. Examples include natural disasters, serious accidents, terrorist acts, war/combat, rape/sexual assault, historical trauma, intimate partner violence, and bullying. People with PTSD have intense, disturbing thoughts and feelings related to their experience that last long after the traumatic event has ended. They may relive the event through flashbacks or nightmares; they may feel sadness, fear, or anger; and they may feel detached or estranged from other people. People with PTSD may avoid situations or people that remind them of the traumatic event, and they may have strong negative reactions to something as ordinary as a loud noise or an accidental touch." American Psychiatric Association, "What Is Posttraumatic Stress Disorder (PTSD)?" January 2, 2023. Physician review by Monica Taylor-Desir, M.D., M.P.H., DFAPA. https://www.psychiatry.org/patients-families/ptsd/what-is-ptsd.

Chapter 4

1. This website, freebythesea.com, is a must-read for anyone dealing with a loved one in active addiction. Dr. Richard Crabbe, "The Three C's of Dealing with an Addict," Free by the Sea Drug and Alcohol Recovery Center, June 1, 2016. https://freebythesea.com/the-three-cs-of-dealing-with-an-addict/.

2. "It should be noted that the 'addiction is a choice' view is largely relegated to individuals and small groups. There are few, if any, nationally recognized substance abuse-focused organizations whose views have not evolved to understanding addiction as a disorder or disease. In fact, the NIH views the idea that addiction is a moral failing as an outdated, ill-informed relic of the past. The American Psychiatric Association (APA) no longer uses 'addiction' as a term or diagnosis. Instead, the APA adopted the phrase 'substance use disorder' as a way to describe problems related to 'compulsive and habitual' substance use. The change was made to avoid confusion surrounding the term addiction, its 'uncertain' definition, and the negative stigma attached to it." Amanda Lautieri and Scot Thomas, "Is Addiction a Disease or a Choice?" American Addiction Centers, September 14, 2022. https://americanaddictioncenters.org/rehab-guide/is-drug-addiction-a-disease.

Chapter 5

1. "The notion that these are 'narcotics' that prevent people from doing intensive therapy when used properly is ridiculous; the converse is true,' says Mark Willenbring, M.D., founder and CEO of Alltyr treatment clinic and former Director of the Division of Treatment and Recovery Research of the National Institute on Alcohol Abuse and Alcoholism at the National Institutes of Health (NIH). In fact, to achieve stable recovery, many people need to stay on these medications for long periods of time—sometimes indefinitely." Leah Walker, "Opioid Addiction: Why Don't More Rehabs Use Suboxone?" American Addition Centers, reviewed by Scot

Thomas, M.D. https://rehabs.com/pro-talk/opioid-addiction-treatment-why-dont-more-rehabs-use-suboxone/, updated February 2, 2023.

2. Thomas R. Kosten and Tony P. George, "The Neurobiology of Opioid Dependence: Implications for Treatment," *Science and Practice Perspectives* 1, no. 1 (July 2022): 13–20. doi: 10.1151/spp021113. PMID: 18567959; PMCID: PMC2851054.

3. "Recent data from 2020 shows that only 13 percent of people with drug use disorders receive any treatment. Only 11 percent of people with opioid use disorder receive one of the three safe and effective medications that could help them quit and stay in recovery." Nora Volkow, "Making Addiction Treatment More Realistic and Pragmatic: The Perfect Should Not Be the Enemy of the Good," National Institute on Drug Abuse, National Institutes of Health, U.S. Department of Health & Human Services, January 4, 2022. https://nida.nih.gov/about-nida/noras-blog/2022/01/making-addiction-treatment-more-realistic-pragmatic-perfect-should-not-be-enemy-good.

4. "Substance Use Disorder (SUD)," Cleveland Clinic. https://my.clevelandclinic.org/health/diseases/16652-drug-addiction-substance-use-disorder-sud, last reviewed October 20, 2022, accessed March 7, 2023.

Chapter 6

1. According to a study done by Frontiers in Psychiatry on the National Institute of Health, "Accumulating evidence shows that exercise influences many of the same signaling molecules and neuroanatomical structures that mediate the positive reinforcing effects of drugs. These studies have revealed that exercise produces protective effects in procedures designed to model different transitional phases that occur during the development of, and recovery from, a substance use disorder." Mark A. Smith and Wendy J. Lynch, "Exercise as a Potential Treatment for Drug Abuse: Evidence from Preclinical Studies," *Frontiers in Psychiatry* 2 (January 12, 2012): 82. doi: 10.3389/fpsyt.2011.00082. PMID: 22347866; PMCID: PMC 3276633. "6 Benefits of Exercise in Addiction Recovery," medically reviewed by Nanci Stockwell, LCSW, MBA, The Recovery Village, last updated May 3, 2022.

2. Katie Richards, "If Cancer Patients Were Treated Like Addicts: Hard-Hitting PSAs Aim to 'Stop the Shame,'" Adweek.com, March 29, 2017. https://www.adweek.com/brand-marketing/if-cancer-patients-were-treated-like-addicts-hard-hitting-psas-aim-to-stop-the-shame/.

3. American Society of Addiction Medicine, "What Is the Definition of Addiction?" https://www.asam.org/quality-care/definition-of-addiction, last updated September 15, 2019.

4. Mayo Clinic, "Post-Traumatic Stress Disorder," December 13, 2022. https://www.mayoclinic.org/diseases-conditions/post-traumatic-stress-disorder/symptoms-causes/syc-20355967.

5. Eric Y. Siu and Tiffany S. Moon, "Opioid-Free and Opioid-Sparing Anesthesia," *International Anesthesiology Clinics* 58, no. 2 (Spring 2020): 34–41. doi: 10.1097/AIA.0000000000000270. https://pubmed.ncbi.nlm.nih.gov/32004171/.

6. National Cancer Institute, "The Genetics of Cancer," National Institutes of Health, August 17, 2022. https://www.cancer.gov/about-cancer/causes-prevention/genetics.

7. Daniel G. Amen, "Drugs and Alcohol Addiction," Amen Clinics, January 1, 2023. https://www.amenclinics.com/conditions/drugs-and-alcohol-addiction/.

8. Pharmaceutical companies play a role in the lack of funding for addiction research. For details, read Lev Facher, "Venture Capital Is Investing Little in New Treatment for Addiction, Report Finds," *Stat News*, February 2, 2023. https://www.statnews.com/2023/02/02/investment-addiction-cures-low-report/.

9. For a more complete understanding of the state of addiction in medical schools, read Jan Hoffman, "Most Doctors Are Ill-Equipped to Deal with the Opioid Epidemic. Few Medical Schools Teach Addiction," *New York Times*, September 10, 2018. https://www.nytimes.com/2018/09/10/health/addiction-medical-schools-treatment.html.

Chapter 7

1. Karla Lopez and Deborah Reed, "Discrimination Against Patients with Substance Use Disorders Remains Prevalent and Harmful: The Case for 42 CFR Part 2," *Health Affairs*, April 30, 2017. https://www.healthaffairs.org/do/10.1377/forefront.20170413.059618/.

2. This article gives statistics regarding the lack of suboxone used as a treatment in hospitals and EDs. Christine Vestal, "Most Hospital ERs Won't Treat Your Addiction. These Will," The Pew Charitable Trusts, September 21, 2018. https://www.pewtrusts.org/en/research-and-analysis/blogs/stateline/2018/09/21/most-hospitalers-wont-treat-your-addiction-these-will.

3. Parvine Sadeghi and James P. Zacny, "Anesthesia Is a Risk Factor for Drug and Alcohol Craving and Relapse in Ex-Abusers," *Med Hypotheses* 53, no. 6 (December 1999): 490–496. doi: 10.1054/mehy.1999.0797. PMID: 10687890. https://pubmed.ncbi.nlm.nih.gov/10687890/.

4. Centers for Disease Control and Prevention, Annual Surveillance Report of Drug-Related Risks and Outcomes United States, January 1, 2018. https://www.cdc.gov/drugoverdose/pdf/pubs/2018-cdc-drug-surveillance-report.pdf.

5. Glenn Murphy and Joseph Szokol, "Use of Methadone in the Perioperative Period," *APSF Newsletter*, February 1, 2018. https://www.apsf.org/article/use-of-methadone-in-the-perioperative-period/.

6. Thomas Kyle Harrison, Howard Kornfeld, Anuj Kailash Aggarwal, and Anna Lembke, "Perioperative Considerations for the Patient with Opioid Use Disorder on Buprenorphine, Methadone, or Naltrexone Maintenance Therapy," *Anesthesiology Clinics* 36, no. 3 (September 2018). doi: 10.1016/j.anclin.2018.04.002. PMID: 30092933.

7. Shabbar I. Ranapurwala, Meghan E. Shanahan, Apostolos A. Alexandridis, Scott K. Proescholdbell, Rebecca B. Naumann, Daniel Edwards, Jr., and Stephen W. Marshall, "Opioid Overdose Mortality Among Former North Carolina Inmates: 2000–2015," *American Journal of Public Health* 108, no. 9 (September 2018): 1207–213. https://doi.org/10.2105/AJPH.2018.304514.

8. Centers for Disease Control and Prevention, "Lifesaving Naloxone," Stop Overdose. https://www.cdc.gov/stopoverdose/naloxone/index.html, last reviewed April 21, 2023.

9. For full instruction on how to plan an intervention, go to Mayo Clinic, "Intervention: Help a Loved One Overcome Addiction," July 20, 2017. https://www.mayoclinic.org/diseases-conditions/mental-illness/in-depth/intervention/art-20047451.

10. David J. Mysels and Maria A. Sullivan, "The Relationship Between Opioid and Sugar Intake: Review of Evidence and Clinical Applications," *Journal of Opioid Management* 6, no. 6 (2010): 445–52. doi:10.5055/jom.2010.0043.

Chapter 8

1. Rajita Sinha, "New Findings on Biological Factors Predicting Addiction Relapse Vulnerability," *Current Psychiatry Reports* 13, no. 5 (October 2011): 398–405. doi: 10.1007/s11920-011-0224-0. PMID: 21792580; PMCID: PMC3674771. https://pubmed.ncbi.nlm.nih.gov/21792580/.

2. These are the guidelines that sobriety houses should follow to ensure safety for their inhabitants as well as the general public. Substance Abuse and Mental Health Service Administration (SAMHSA), "Recovery Housing: Best Practices and Suggested Guidelines," U.S. Department of Health & Human Services. https://www.samhsa.gov/resource/ebp/recovery-housing-best-practices-suggested-guidelines.

3. Though kratom tea is legal, there are safety concerns regarding it and other kratom-based products, which have made some people wary about using it. This article explores kratom tea, including its effects, safety, and risks. Ryan Raman, "What Is Kratom Tea, and Is It Safe?" *Healthline Newsletter*, February 27, 2020. Medically reviewed by Jillian Kubala, MS, RD. https://www.healthline.com/nutrition/kratom-tea.

4. This study gives statistics backing up the fact that many doctors and media staff have a prejudice against those with SUD. Brandon Muncan, Suzan M. Walters, Jerel Ezell, and Danielle C. Ompad, "'They look

at us like junkies': Influences of Drug Use Stigma on the Healthcare Engagement of People Who Inject Drugs in New York City," *Harm Reduction Journal* 17, article 53 (July 31, 2020). doi: 10.1186/s12954-020-00399-8. PMID: 32736624; PMCID: PMC7393740.

5. "'There have been a lot of anecdotal reports suggesting kratom has some pain-relieving properties and has helped transition users from prescription opioids to this product,' said Chris McCurdy, Ph.D., a professor of medicinal chemistry in the UF College of Pharmacy. 'Scientifically, this becomes one of the most important kratom studies released showing support as a potential treatment option for opioid withdrawal syndrome or opioid use disorder.'" Edward W. Boyer, Kavita M. Babu, Jessica E. Adkins, Christopher R. McCurdy, and John H. Halpern, "Self-Treatment of Opioid Withdrawal Using Kratom (*Mitragynia speciosa korth*)," *Addiction* 103, no. 6 (June 2008): 1048–050. doi: 10.1111/j.1360-0443.2008.02209.x. PMID: 18482427; PMCID: PMC3670991. https://www.ncbi.nlm.nih.gov/pmc/articles/PMC3670991/.

6. Nina Feldman, "Many 'Recovery Houses' Won't Let Residents Use Medicine to Quit Opioids," NPR, September 12, 2018. https://www.npr.org/sections/health-shots/2018/09/12/644685850/many-recovery-houses-wont-let-residents-use-medicine-to-quit-opioids.

7. "AA's success rate has been historically difficult to measure, largely because the program is anonymous. But thanks to rigorous research done by John F. Kelly, Keith Humphreys, and Marica Ferri, we now know that Alcoholics Anonymous and clinically-related Twelve-Step Facilitation programs can be just as, or more effective than treatment modalities like Cognitive Behavioral Therapy (CBT) to maintain long-term sobriety for people with alcohol use disorder." Marla Kauffman, "Alcoholics Anonymous Works. But It's Important to Give People Options When It Comes to Recovery," IRETA, June 16, 2022. ttps://ireta.org/alcoholics-anonymous-works-but-its-important-to-give-people-options-when-it-comes-to-recovery/.

8. Andrew Rosen, "Not All Addicts Are Alike," Center for Treatment of Anxiety and Mood Disorders. https://centerforanxietydisorders.com/not-addicts-alike/.

9. "This study investigated the client's perceptions of his lived experience of various treatment approaches and whether or not recovery program professionals made flexible adjustments to incorporate best practices and adjust for the needs and obstacles specific to the individual client in treatment planning and execution." Rose M. Valero, "Hearing the Voice of Addiction: A Case Study," doctoral dissertation, California Institute of Integral Studies, 2021 (Publication No. 28497929). ProQuest, https://www.proquest.com/openview/14fcc88025b72c30823eae8377b1f644/1?pq-origsite=gscholar&cbl=18750&diss=y.

10. This website details dual diagnosis/co-occurring conditions. Some include anxiety and mood disorders, schizophrenia, bipolar disorder, major depressive disorder, conduct disorders, post-traumatic stress disorder, and attention deficit hyperactivity disorder. No specific combinations of mental and substance use disorders are defined uniquely as co-occurring disorders. SAMHSA, "Co-Occurring Disorders and Other Health Conditions," U.S. Department of Health & Human Services. https://www.samhsa.gov/medications-substance-use-disorders/medications-counseling-related-conditions/co-occurring-disorders, last updated July 26, 2023.

11. Khodadad Namiranian, Jonathan Siglin, John David Sorkin, Edward J. Norris, Minu Aghevli, and Edward C. Covington, "Postoperative Opioid Misuse in Patients with Opioid Use Disorders Maintained on Opioid Agonist Treatment," *Journal of Substance Abuse Treatment* 109 (February 2020): 8–13. doi: 10.1016/j.jsat.2019.10.007. Epub 2019 Oct 31. PMID: 31856954; PMCID: PMC7416727.

12. Mimi O'Donnell as told to Adam Green, "Mimi O'Donnell Reflects on the Loss of Philip Seymour Hoffman and the Devastation of Addiction," *Vogue*, December 13, 2017. https://www.vogue.com/article/philip-seymour-hoffman-mimi-odonnell-vogue-january-2018-issue.

13. Sarah E. Wakeman, Marc R. Larochelle, Omid Ameli, et al., "Comparative Effectiveness of Different Treatment

Pathways for Opioid Use Disorder," *JAMA Network Open* 3, no. 2 (February 5, 2020):e1920622. doi:10.1001/jamanetworkopen.2019.20622.

14. This website gives details about the medications that have been approved by the U.S. Food and Drug Administration (FDA) to assist with the treatment of substance use disorders, a process known as Medication-Assisted Treatment. Jessica Miller, "Medication-Assisted Treatment," Addictionhelp.com, May 24, 2022. Medically reviewed by Kent S. Hoffman. https://www.addictionhelp.com/drug-rehab/medication-assisted-treatment/.

15. "Cravings are not all the same, nor do they elicit the same neurological reactions." Raymond F. Anton, "What Is Craving? Models and Implications for Treatment," *Alcohol Research & Health* 23, no. 3 (1999): 165–73. PMID: 10890811; PMCID: PMC6760371. https://www.ncbi.nlm.nih.gov/pmc/articles/PMC6760371/.

16. Mansi Shah and Martin R. Huecker, "Opioid Withdrawal," *StatPearls*, January 2023. Available from https://www.ncbi.nlm.nih.gov/books/NBK526012/, last updated July 21, 2023.

17. Taylor Bennett, "What Does Addiction Feel Like? Here's a Clear Picture of What It's Like to Experience Addiction, to Go Through Withdrawal, and to Work Toward Sobriety," Thriveworks, August 10, 2018. Clinically reviewed by Emily Simonian, M.A., LMFT. https://thriveworks.com/blog/experience-addiction-withdrawal-sobriety/.

18. National Institute of Diabetes and Digestive and Kidney Diseases, "About the Special Diabetes Program." https://www.niddk.nih.gov/about-niddk/research-areas/diabetes/type-1-diabetes-special-statutory-funding-program/about-special-diabetes-program.

19. "The High Price of the Opioid Crisis, 2021," The Pew Charitable Trusts, August 27, 2021. https://www.pewtrusts.org/en/research-and-analysis/data-visualizations/2021/the-high-price-of-the-opioid-crisis-2021.

Chapter 9

1. The following article gives a scientific breakdown of how exercise can help keep sobriety. Wendy J. Lynch, Alexis B. Peterson, Victoria Sanchez, Jean Abel, and Mark A. Smith, "Exercise as a Novel Treatment for Drug Addiction: A Neurobiological and Stage-Dependent Hypothesis," *Neuroscience Biobehavioral Reviews* 37, no. 8 (September 2013): 1622–644. doi: 10.1016/j.neubiorev.2013.06.011. PMID: 23806439; PMCID: PMC3788047. https://www.ncbi.nlm.nih.gov/pmc/articles/PMC3788047/.

2. Stephanie Watson, "Feel-Good Hormones: How They Affect Your Mind, Mood, and Body," Harvard Health, July 20, 2021. https://www.health.harvard.edu/mind-and-mood/feel-good-hormones-how-they-affect-your-mind-mood-and-body.

3. Ream Al-Hasani and Michael R. Bruchas, "Molecular Mechanisms of Opioid Receptor-Dependent Signaling and Behavior," *Anesthesiology* 115, no. 6 (2011):1363–381. doi:://www.ncbi.nlm.nih.gov/pmc/articles/PMC3698859/.

4. According to the American Psychiatric Association, "PTSD can occur in all people of any ethnicity, nationality, or culture and at any age. PTSD affects approximately 3.5 percent of U.S. adults every year, and an estimated one in 11 people will be diagnosed with PTSD in their lifetime. Women are twice as likely as men to have PTSD. Three ethnic groups: U.S. Latinos, African Americans, and American Indians are disproportionately affected and have higher rates of PTSD than non–Latino whites." https://www.psychiatry.org/patients-families/ptsd/what-is-ptsd. "PTSD is a disorder in which a person has difficulty recovering after experiencing or witnessing a terrifying event. The condition may last months or years, with triggers that can bring back memories of the trauma accompanied by intense emotional and physical reactions." Georgia Hope. https://gahope.org/post-traumatic-stress-disorder-ptsd-awareness.

5. John Hudak, "The Farm Bill, Hemp Legalization and the Status of CBD: An Explainer," The Brookings Institution, December 13, 2018. https://www.brookings.edu/blog/fixgov/2018/12/14/the-farm-bill-hemp-and-cbd-explainer.

6. Esther M. Blessing, Maria M. Steenkamp, Jorge Manzanares, and Charles

R. Marmar, "Cannabidiol as a Potential Treatment for Anxiety Disorders," *Neurotherapeutics* 12, no. 4 (October 2015): 825–836. doi: 10.1007/s13311-015-0387-1. PMID: 26341731; PMCID: PMC4604171.

7. "Hemp CBD Market to Reach $16 Billion by 2025," Brightfield, January 1, 2018. https://blog.brightfieldgroup.com/hemp-cbd-market-size.

8. Shaklee, "The Shaklee Difference—Organic and Beyond," Shaklee.com, January 1, 2023. https://us.shaklee.com/about-us.

Chapter 10

1. Falling "in love" is often the chemical reaction called limerance. For a full breakdown of limerance, read the article by "Dr. L," "The Neuroscience of Limerence," Living with Limerence, October 3, 2020. https://livingwithlimerence.com/the-neuroscience-of-limerence/.

2. Centers for Disease Control and Prevention, "Drug Overdose Deaths in the U.S. Top 100,000 Annually," National Center for Health Statistics, November 17, 2021. https://www.cdc.gov/nchs/pressroom/nchs_press_releases/2021/20211117.htm.

3. Barbara Ferrer, Data Report: Accidental Drug Overdose Deaths in Los Angeles County During the COIVD-19 Pandemic, Public Health LA County, January 1, 2021. http://publichealth.lacounty.gov/sapc/MDU/SpecialReport/AccidentalDrugOverdoseReport.pdf.

4. Alan K. Davis, Frederick S. Barrett, Darrick G. May, Mary P. Cosimano, Nathan D. Sepeda, Matthew W. Johnson, Patrick H. Finan, and Roland R. Griffiths, "Effects of Psilocybin-Assisted Therapy on Major Depressive Disorder: A Randomized Clinical Trial," *JAMA Psychiatry* 78, no. 5 (May 1, 2021): 481–489. doi: 10.1001/jamapsychiatry.2020.3285.

Erratum in *JAMA Psychiatry* 78, no. 5 (February 10, 2021). PMID: 33146667; PMCID: PMC7643046.

5. Alcohol and Drug Foundation, "LSD as a Therapeutic Treatment," July 19, 2018. https://adf.org.au/insights/lsd-therapeutic-treatment/.

6. Sherwin Nuland, "Sigmund Freud's Cocaine Years," *The New York Times*, July 21, 2011. https://www.nytimes.com/2011/07/24/books/review/an-anatomy-of-addiction-by-howard-markel-book-review.html.

7. Susan M. Stine and T.R. Kosten, "Reduction of Opiate Withdrawal-Like Symptoms by Cocaine Abuse During Methadone and Buprenorphine Maintenance," *American Journal of Drug and Alcohol Abuse* 20, no. 4 (November 1994): 445–58. doi: 10.3109/00952299409109183. PMID: 7832179. https://pubmed.ncbi.nlm.nih.gov/7832179/.

8. "Exclusive: Could Innovative Brain Surgery Be the Tool to Treat Severe Substance Abuse?" NBC News, September 29, 2021. https://www.nbcnews.com/nightly-news/video/exclusive-could-innovative-brain-surgery-be-tool-to-treat-severe-substance-abuse-122328645783.

9. Marco Diana, "The Dopamine Hypothesis of Drug Addiction and Its Potential Therapeutic Value," *Frontiers in Psychiatry* 2, 64 (November 29, 2011). doi:10.3389/fpsyt.2011.00064.

Chapter 11

1. Emma Jane Rose, Giorgia Picci, and Diana H. Fishbein, "Neurocognitive Precursors of Substance Misuse Corresponding to Risk, Resistance, and Resilience Pathways: Implications for Prevention Science," *Frontiers in Society* 10, June 14, 2019. https://www.frontiersin.org/articles/10.3389/fpsyt.2019.00399/full.

Bibliography

"Adderall Neurotoxicity from Misuse." Oxford Treatment Center, updated May 23, 2023. https://oxfordtreatment.com/prescription-drug-abuse/adderall/neurotoxicity/.
Akpan, Nsikan, and Julia Griffin. "How a Brain Gets Hooked on Opioids." *PBS News Hour*, October 9, 2017. https://www.pbs.org/newshour/science/brain-gets-hooked-opioids.
Al-Hasani, Ream, and Michael R. Bruchas. "Molecular Mechanisms of Opioid Receptor-Dependent Signaling and Behavior." *Anesthesiology* 115, no. 6 (2011): 1363–381. doi:://www.ncbi.nlm.nih.gov/pmc/articles/PMC3698859/.
Alcohol and Drug Foundation. "LSD as a Therapeutic Treatment." July 19, 2018. https://adf.org.au/insights/lsd-therapeutic-treatment/.
Amen, Daniel G. "Drugs and Alcohol Addiction." Amen Clinics, accessed January 1, 2023. https://www.amenclinics.com/conditions/drugs-and-alcohol-addiction/.
Amen, Daniel G., and David E. Smith. "Unchain Your Brain." Dr. David E. Smith, accessed March 13, 2022. http://www.drdave.org/Unchain-Your-Brain.
American Addiction Centers. "Common Side Effects of Suboxone (Buprenorphine/Naloxone)." January 10, 2022, last updated September 7, 2022. https://americanaddictioncenters.org/suboxone/side-effects.
American Psychiatric Association. "What Is Posttraumatic Stress Disorder (PTSD)?" Pschiatry.org, accessed January 2, 2023. https://www.psychiatry.org/patients-families/ptsd/what-is-ptsd.
American Society of Addiction Medicine. *The ASAM National Practice Guideline for the Use of Medications in the Treatment of Addiction Involving Opioid Use*. National Institute on Drug Abuse. January 2018. https://www.asam.org/docs/default-source/practice-support/guidelines-and-consensus-docs/asam-national-practice-guideline-pocketguide.pdf.
American Society of Addiction Medicine. "More Training Needed to Address Addiction Workforce Shortage: Congress Should Fund Authorized Demonstration Program at HRSA in FY20." Accessed March 24, 2022. https://www.asam.org/docs/default-source/advocacy/asam-training-demo-one-pagerb1ff289472bc604ca5b7ff000030b21a.pdf?sfvrsn=264348c2_2.
American Society of Addiction Medicine. "What Is the Definition of Addiction?" Updated September 15, 2019. https://www.asam.org/quality-care/definition-of-addiction.
American Society of Anesthesiologists. "Opioid Abuse: Statistics, Signs & Symptoms—Made for This Moment." Accessed March 24, 2022. https://www.asahq.org/madeforthismoment/pain-management/opioid-treatment/opioid-abuse/.
Anton, Raymond F. "What Is Craving? Models and Implications for Treatment." *Alcohol Research & Health* 23, no. 3 (1999): 165–73. PMID: 10890811; PMCID: PMC6760371. https://www.ncbi.nlm.nih.gov/pmc/articles/PMC6760371/.
Baksh, Justin. "Do Other Countries Treat Addiction Like Us and See It as a Global Disease?" Foundations Wellness Center, October 7, 2019. https://www.foundationswellness.net/drug-abuse/do-other-countries-treat-addiction-like-us-and-see-it-as-a-global-disease/.

Bennett, Taylor. "What Does Addiction Feel Like? Here's a Clear Picture of What It's Like to Experience Addiction, to Go Through Withdrawal, and to Work Toward Sobriety." Thriveworks, August 10, 2018. Clinically reviewed by Emily Simonian, M.A., LMFT. https://thriveworks.com/blog/experience-addiction-withdrawal-sobriety/.

Bettinger, Jeffrey J., Jeffrey Fundin, and Charles E. Argoff. "Buprenorphine and Surgery: What's the Protocol?" Practical Pain Management, April 29, 2019. https://www.practicalpainmanagement.com/resource-centers/opioid-monitoring-2nd-ed/buprenorphine-surgery-what-protocol.

Billey, Rep. Tom (R–VA–7). H.R.2634–106th Congress (1999–2000). Drug Addiction Treatment Act of 2000. July 27, 2000. https://www.congress.gov/bill/106th-congress/house-bill/2634.

Blessing, Esther M., Maria M. Steenkamp, Jorge Manzanares, and Charles R. Marmar. "Cannabidiol as a Potential Treatment for Anxiety Disorders." *Neurotherapeutics* 12, no. 4 (October 2015): 825–36. doi: 10.1007/s13311-015-0387-1. PMID: 26341731; PMCID: PMC4604171.

Boyer, Edward W., Kavita M. Babu, Jessica E. Adkins, Christopher R. McCurdy, and John H. Halpern. "Self-Treatment of Opioid Withdrawal Using Kratom (*Mitragynia speciosa korth*)." *Addiction* 103, no. 6 (June 2008): 1048–050. doi: 10.1111/j.1360-0443.2008.02209.x. PMID: 18482427; PMCID: PMC3670991. https://www.ncbi.nlm.nih.gov/pmc/articles/PMC3670991/.

Burns, Jamie A., Danielle S. Kroll, Dana E. Feldman, Christopher Kure Liu, Peter Manza, Corine E. Wiers, Nora D. Volkow, and Gene-Jack Wang. "Molecular Imaging of Opioid and Dopamine Systems: Insights into the Pharmacogenetics of Opioid Use Disorders." *Frontiers in Psychiatry*, September 18, 2019. https://www.frontiersin.org/articles/10.3389/fpsyt.2019.00626/full.

Bydlowska, Jowita. "Are You Really Sober If You're on Meds?" The Fix, January 3, 2019. https://www.thefix.com/content/are-you-really-sober-if-youre-meds.

Carmona, Melissa. "Alcohol Relapse Rates & Abstinence Statistics." The Recovery Village Drug and Alcohol Rehab, updated July 28, 2022. https://www.therecoveryvillage.com/alcohol-abuse/related-topics/alcohol-relapse-statistics/.

Centers for Disease Control and Prevention. Annual Surveillance Report of Drug-Related Risks and Outcomes United States. January 1, 2018. https://www.cdc.gov/drugoverdose/pdf/pubs/2018-cdc-drug-surveillance-report.pdf.

Centers for Disease Control and Prevention. "Drug Overdose Deaths in the U.S. Top 100,000 Annually." National Center for Health Statistics, November 17, 2021. https://www.cdc.gov/nchs/pressroom/nchs_press_releases/2021/20211117.htm.

Centers for Disease Control and Prevention. "Lifesaving Naloxone." Stop Overdose, last reviewed April 21, 2023. https://www.cdc.gov/stopoverdose/naloxone/index.html.

Chakradhar, Shraddha, and Casey Ross. "The History of OxyContin, Told Through Unsealed Purdue Documents." STAT, December 3, 2019. https://www.statnews.com/2019/12/03/oxycontin-history-told-through-purdue-pharma-documents/.

Chant, Ian. "LSD May Cure Some Addicts." *Scientific American*, July 1, 2012. https://www.scientificamerican.com/article/lsd-may-cure-some-addicts/.

Clavel, Alfred, Jr., M.D. "5 Ways Opioids and Their Negative Side Effects Make Your Pain Worse." Health Partners, accessed January 1, 2023. https://www.healthpartners.com/blog/why-opioids-make-pain-worse/.

"Controversy Over DSM-5: New Mental Health Guide." *Nursing Times*, August 24, 2013. https://www.nursingtimes.net/news/behind-the-headlines/controversy-over-dsm-5-new-mental-health-guide-24-08-2013/.

Crabbe, Dr. Richard. "The Three C's of Dealing with an Addict." Free by the Sea Drug and Alcohol Recovery Center, June 1, 2016. https://freebythesea.com/the-three-cs-of-dealing-with-an-addict/.

Davis, Alan K., Frederick S. Barrett, Darrick G. May, Mary P. Cosimano, Nathan D. Sepeda, Matthew W. Johnson, Patrick H. Finan, and Roland R. Griffiths. "Effects of Psilocybin-Assisted Therapy on Major Depressive Disorder: A Randomized Clinical Trial." *JAMA Psychiatry* 78, no. 5 (May 1, 2021): 481–489. doi: 10.1001/

jamapsychiatry.2020.3285. Erratum in *JAMA Psychiatry* 78, no. 5 (February 10, 2021). PMID: 33146667; PMCID: PMC7643046.

Diana, Marco. "The Dopamine Hypothesis of Drug Addiction and Its Potential Therapeutic Value." *Frontiers in Psychiatry* 2, 64 (November 29, 2011). doi:10.3389/fpsyt.2011.00064.

"Dr. L." "The Neuroscience of Limerence." Living with Limerence, October 3, 2020. https://livingwithlimerence.com/the-neuroscience-of-limerence/.

"Dopamine Burnout: Dopamine Deficiency Symptoms & Addiction." AspenRidge, March 29, 2021. https://www.aspenridgerecoverycenters.com/dopamine-burnout/.

Effatpanah, Mohammad, Mahdi Rezaei, Hosein Effatpanah, Zeynab Effatpanah, Hamed Kord Varkaneh, Seyed Mohammad Mousavi, Somaye Fatahi, Giulia Rinaldi, and Rezvan Hashemi. "Magnesium Status and Attention Deficit Hyperactivity Disorder (ADHD): A Meta-Analysis." *Psychiatry Research* 274 (April 2019): 228–234. https://www.sciencedirect.com/science/article/abs/pii/S0165178118318456.

El-Malhany, Nadia, Mariangela Gulisano, Renata Rizzo, and Paolo Curatolo. "Tourette Syndrome and Comorbid ADHD: Causes and Consequences." *European Journal of Pediatrics* 174, no. 3 (March 2015): 279–288. doi: 10.1007/s00431-014-2417-0. PMID: 25224657.

Erikson, Mandy. "Alcoholics Anonymous Most Effective Path to Alcohol Abstinence." Stanford Medicine, March 11, 2020. https://med.stanford.edu/news/all-news/2020/03/alcoholics-anonymous-most-effective-path-to-alcohol-abstinence.html.

"Exclusive: Could Innovative Brain Surgery Be the Tool to Treat Severe Substance Abuse?" NBC News, September 29, 2021. https://www.nbcnews.com/nightly-news/video/exclusive-could-innovative-brain-surgery-be-tool-to-treat-severe-substance-abuse-122328645783.

Ezquerra-Romano, I. Ivan, Will Lawn, E. Krupitsky, and Celia Morgan. "Ketamine for the Treatment of Addiction: Evidence and Potential Mechanisms." *Neuropharmacology* 142 (November 2018): 72–82. https://www.sciencedirect.com/science/article/abs/pii/S0028390818300170.

Fatcher, Lev. "Venture Capital Is Investing Little in New Treatment for Addiction, Report Finds." *Stat News*, February 2, 2023. https://www.statnews.com/2023/02/02/investment-addiction-cures-low-report/.

Feduccia, Allison A., Julie Holland, and Michael C. Mithoefer. "Progress and Promise for the MDMA Drug Development Program" *Psychopharmacology* 235, no. 2 (February 2018). https://pubmed.ncbi.nlm.nih.gov/29152674/.

Feldman, Nina. "Many 'Recovery Houses' Won't Let Residents Use Medicine to Quit Opioids." NPR, September 12, 2018. https://www.npr.org/sections/health-shots/2018/09/12/644685850/many-recovery-houses-wont-let-residents-use-medicine-to-quit-opioids.

Ferrer, Barbara. Data Report: Accidental Drug Overdose Deaths in Los Angeles County During the COIVD-19 Pandemic, Public Health LA County, January 1, 2021. http://publichealth.lacounty.gov/sapc/MDU/SpecialReport/AccidentalDrugOverdoseReport.pdf.

Gant, C. "The 6 Amino Acids Necessary to Alleviate Your Cravings." National Integrated Health Associated, accessed March 24, 2022. https://www.nihadc.com/library/dr-chas-gant/144-summation-of-the-6-essential-amino-acids-needed-to-alleviate-your-cravings-rev/file.html?accept_license=1.

Glaser, Gabrielle. "The Irrationality of Alcoholics Anonymous." *The Atlantic*, April 2015. https://www.theatlantic.com/magazine/archive/2015/04/the-irrationality-of-alcoholics-anonymous/386255/.

Gupta, Arun, M.D. *The Preventable Epidemic: A Frontline Doctor's Experience and Recommendations to Resolve America's Opioid Crisis*, 1st ed. Monroe, MI: RAOE Foundation, 2022. https://doi.org/979-8985477603.

Handberg, Roger B. "The Opioid Epidemic in Florida: 2000 to 2017." The Florida Bar, May 2020. https://www.floridabar.org/the-florida-bar-journal/the-opioid-epidemic-in-florida-2000-to-2017/.

Hardee, Jillian. "Science Says: Addiction Is a Chronic Disease, Not a Moral Failing."

Michigan Medicine, University of Michigan, May 19, 2017. https://healthblog.uofmhealth.org/brain-health/science-says-addiction-a-chronic-disease-not-a-moral-failing.

Harrison, Thomas Kyle, Howard Kornfeld, Anuj Kailash Aggarwal, and Anna Lembky. "Perioperative Considerations for the Patient with Opioid Use Disorder on Buprenorphine, Methadone, or Naltrexone Maintenance Therapy." *Anesthesiology Clinics* 36, no. 3 (September 2018). doi:10.1016/j.anclin.2018.04.002. PMID: 30092933.

Harvard School of Public Health. "Cost of Diabetes Hits 825 Billion Dollars a Year." June 22, 2018. https://www.hsph.harvard.edu/news/press-releases/diabetes-cost-825-billion-a-year.

Hemamy, Mostafa, Naseh Pahlavani, Alireza Amanollahi, Sheikh Mohammed Shriful Islam, Jenna McVicar, Gholamreza Askari, and Mahsa Malekahmadi. "The Effect of Vitamin D and Magnesium Supplementation on the Mental Health Status of Attention-Deficit Hyperactive Children: A Randomized Controlled Trial." *BMC Pediatrics* 21, no. 1 (April 17, 2021): 178. doi: 10.1186/s12887-021-02631-1.

"Hemp CBD Market to Reach $16 Billion by 2025." Brightfield, January 1, 2018. https://blog.brightfieldgroup.com/hemp-cbd-market-size.

"The High Price of the Opioid Crisis, 2021." The Pew Charitable Trusts, August 27, 2021. https://www.pewtrusts.org/en/research-and-analysis/data-visualizations/2021/the-high-price-of-the-opioid-crisis-2021.

Hoffman, Jan. "Most Doctors Are Ill-Equipped to Deal with the Opioid Epidemic. Few Medical Schools Teach Addiction." *New York Times*, September 10, 2018. https://www.nytimes.com/2018/09/10/health/addiction-medical-schools-treatment.html.

"How Long Does It Take the Brain to Recover from Addiction?" StoneRidge: Center for Brains, January 27, 2022. https://pronghornpsych.com/how-long-for-the-brain-to-recover-from-addiction/.

Hudak, John. "The Farm Bill, Hemp Legalization and the Status of CBD: An Explainer." The Brookings Institution, December 13, 2018. https://www.brookings.edu/blog/fixgov/2018/12/14/the-farm-bill-hemp-and-cbd-explainer.

Itin, Constantin, Dinorah Barasch, Abraham J. Domb, and Amnon Hoffman. "Prolonged Oral Transmucosal Delivery of Highly Lipophilic Drug Cannabidiol." *International Journal of Pharmaceutics* 581 (May 15, 2020). https://www.sciencedirect.com/science/article/abs/pii/S037851732030260X?via%3Dihu.

Jerome, Lisa, Shira Schuster, and B. Berra Yazar-Klosinski. "Can MDMA Play a Role in the Treatment of Substance Abuse?" *Current Drug Abuse Reviews* 6, no. 1 (March 6, 2013): 54–62. https://pubmed.ncbi.nlm.nih.gov/23627786/.

Johns Hopkins Medicine. "Psychedelic Treatment with Psilocybin Relieves Major Depression, a Study shows." Johns Hopkins Medicine Newsroom, November 4, 2020. https://www.hopkinsmedicine.org/news/newsroom/news-releases/psychedelic-treatment-with-psilocybin-relieves-major-depression-study-shows.

Juergens, Jeffrey. "Addiction." Addiction Center, March 9, 2022, last edited April 17, 2023. https://www.addictioncenter.com/addiction/.

Kauffman, Marla. "Alcoholics Anonymous Works. But It's Important to Give People Options When It Comes to Recovery." IRETA, June 16, 2022. tps://ireta.org/alcoholics-anonymous-works-but-its-important-to-give-people-options-when-it-comes-to-recovery/.

Kosten, Thomas R., and Tony P. George. "The Neurobiology of Opioid Dependence: Implications for Treatment." *Science and Practice Perspectives* 1, no. 1 (July 2022): 13–20. doi: 10.1151/spp021113. PMID: 18567959; PMCID: PMC2851054.

"Kratom and Suboxone: Everything You Need to Know." Bicycle Health, accessed May 11, 2022. Medically reviewed by Elene Hill, M.D., MPH. https://www.bicyclehealth.com/blog/kratom-suboxone-everything-you-need-to-know.

Krupitsky, Evgeny, Andrey Burakov, Tatyana Romanova, Igor Dunaevsky, Rick Strassman, and Alexander Grinenko. "Ketamine Psychotherapy for Heroin Addiction: Immediate Effects and Two-Year Follow-Up." Journal of Substance Abuse Treatment 23, no. 4 (December 2022): 273–283. https://www.sciencedirect.com/science/article/abs/pii/S0740547202002751.

Lasagna, Louis. "The Hippocratic Oath: Modern Version." *Nova*, January 1, 1964. https://www.pbs.org/wgbh/nova/doctors/oath_modern.html.
Lautieri, Amanda, and Scot Thomas. "Is Addiction a Disease or a Choice?" American Addiction Centers, September 14, 2022. https://americanaddictioncenters.org/rehab-guide/is-drug-addiction-a-disease.
Levran, Orna, Vadim Yuferov, and Mary Jeanne Kreek. "The Genetics of the Opioid System and Specific Drug Addictions." *Human Genetics* 131, no. 6 (June 2012): 823–842. doi: 10.1007/s00439-012-1172-4. PMID: 22547174; PMCID: PMC3721349.
Levreau, Dawn M. "Quality Healthcare, Public Trust, and Setting the Standards in Addiction Medicine: Science, Skill, and Compassion." American Board of Addiction Medicine, accessed March 24, 2022. https://www.abam.net/.
Lochran, Michael, and Laura Cavanagh. "The Neurobiology of Addiction—Part Two: Relapse, Abstinence, and Treatment." *Renascent*, April 23, 2021. https://renascent.ca/the-neurobiology-of-addiction-part-two-relapse-abstinence-and-treatment/.
Lopez, German. "A Rising Death Toll." *New York Times*, February 13, 2022. https://www.nytimes.com/2022/02/13/briefing/opioids-drug-overdose-death-toll.html.
Lopez, Karla, and Deborah Reed. "Discrimination Against Patients with Substance Use Disorders Remains Prevalent and Harmful: The Case for 42 CFR Part 2." *Health Affairs*, April 30, 2017. https://www.healthaffairs.org/do/10.1377/forefront.20170413.059618/.
Lynch, Shalini S., PharmD. "Tolerance and Resistance to Drugs." *Merck Manual Online*, full review/revision July 2022, modified September 2022. https://www.merckmanuals.com/home/drugs/factors-affecting-response-to-drugs/tolerance-and-resistance-to-drugs.
Lynch, Wendy J., Alexis B. Peterson, Victoria Sanchez, Jean Abel, and Mark A. Smith. "Exercise as a Novel Treatment for Drug Addiction: A Neurobiological and Stage-Dependent Hypothesis." *Neuroscience Biobehavioral Reviews* 37, no. 8 (September 2013): 1622–644. doi: 10.1016/j.neubiorev.2013.06.011. PMID: 23806439; PMCID: PMC3788047. https://www.ncbi.nlm.nih.gov/pmc/articles/PMC3788047/.
"Magnesium Shown to Calm Hyperactivity in Children." E.I.N. Newswires, September 30, 2022. https://www.einnews.com/pr_news/592794090/magnesium-shown-to-calm-hyperactivity-in-children.
Marston-Salem, Natalie. "Mental Health Awareness Month: Is Addiction a Mental Illness?" Fountain Hills Recovery, accessed October 15, 2021. https://www.fountainhillsrecovery.com/blog/mental-health-awareness-month/.
Matuszak, Pat. "Treating Addiction Like Any Other Disease." Cumberland Hall Hospital, May 22, 2018. https://www.cumberlandhallhospital.com/2018/05/22/treating-addiction-like-disease/.
Mayo Clinic. "Intervention: Help a Loved One Overcome Addiction." July 20, 2017. https://www.mayoclinic.org/diseases-conditions/mental-illness/in-depth/intervention/art-20047451.
Mayo Clinic. "Post-Traumatic Stress Disorder." December 13, 2022. https://www.mayoclinic.org/diseases-conditions/post-traumatic-stress-disorder/symptoms-causes/syc-20355967.
Mayo Foundation for Medical Education and Research. "Drug Addiction (Substance Use Disorder)." Mayo Clinic, October 26, 2017. https://www.mayoclinic.org/diseases-conditions/drug-addiction/symptoms-causes/syc-20365112.
Miller, Jessica. "Medication-Assisted Treatment." Addictionhelp.com, May 24, 2022. Medically reviewed by Kent S. Hoffman. https://www.addictionhelp.com/drug-rehab/medication-assisted-treatment/.
Miron, Jeffrey, Greg Sollenberger, and Laura Nicolae. "Overdosing on Regulation: How Government Caused the Opioid Epidemic." Cato.org, February 14, 2029. https://www.cato.org/policy-analysis/overdosing-regulation-how-government-caused-opioid-epidemic#summary-and-policy-implications.
Moawad, Heidi. "Ketamine Is an Anesthetic Medication for Surgery." Verywell Health, October 1, 2020, updated July 20, 2022. Medically reviewed by David Hampton, M.D. https://www.verywellhealth.com/ketamine-5077592.
Muncan, Brandon, Suzan M. Walters, Jerel Ezell, and Danielle C. Ompad. "'They look at

us like junkies': Influences of Drug Use Stigma on the Healthcare Engagement of People Who Inject Drugs in New York City." *Harm Reduction Journal* 17, article 53 (July 31, 2020). doi: 10.1186/s12954-020-00399-8. PMID: 32736624; PMCID: PMC7393740.

Murphy, Glenn, and Joseph Szokol. "Use of Methadone in the Perioperative Period." *APSF Newsletter*, February 1, 2018. https://www.apsf.org/article/use-of-methadone-in-the-perioperative-period/.

Mysels, David J., and Maria A. Sullivan. "The Relationship Between Opioid and Sugar Intake: Review of Evidence and Clinical Applications." *Journal of Opioid Management* 6, no. 6 (2010): 445–52. doi:10.5055/jom.2010.0043.

Namiranian, Khodadad, Jonathan Siglin, John David Sorkin, Edward J. Norris, Minu Aghevli, and Edward C. Covington. "Postoperative Opioid Misuse in Patients with Opioid Use Disorders Maintained on Opioid Agonist Treatment." *Journal of Substance Abuse Treatment* 109 (February 2020): 8–13. doi: 10.1016/j.jsat.2019.10.007. Epub 2019 Oct 31. PMID: 31856954; PMCID: PMC7416727.

National Cancer Institute. "The Genetics of Cancer." National Institutes of Health, August 17, 2022. https://www.cancer.gov/about-cancer/causes-prevention/genetics.

National Institute of Diabetes and Digestive and Kidney Diseases. "About the Special Diabetes Program." https://www.niddk.nih.gov/about-niddk/research-areas/diabetes/type-1-diabetes-special-statutory-funding-program/about-special-diabetes-program

National Institute on Drug Abuse. "Co-Prescribing Opioids and Benzodiazepines." National Institutes of Health, U.S. Department of Health & Human Services, November 7, 2022. https://nida.nih.gov/research-topics/opioids/benzodiazepines-opioids.

National Institute on Drug Abuse. "Drug Overdose Death Rates." National Institutes of Health, U.S. Department of Health & Human Services, February 9, 2019. https://nida.nih.gov/research-topics/trends-statistics/overdose-death-rates.

National Institute on Drug Abuse. "Drugs and the Brain." National Institutes of Health, U.S. Department of Health & Human Services, March 22, 2022. https://nida.nih.gov/publications/drugs-brains-behavior-science-addiction/drugs-brain.

National Institute on Drug Abuse. "Prescription Stimulants DrugFacts." National Institutes of Health, U.S. Department of Health & Human Services, June 2018. https://nida.nih.gov/publications/drugfacts/prescription-stimulants.

Nowacka, Agata, and Malgorzata Borczyk. "Ketamine Applications Beyond Anesthesia—A Literature Review." *European Journal of Pharmacology* 860 (October 2019). https://www.sciencedirect.com/science/article/abs/pii/S0014299919304996.

Nuland, Sherwin. "Sigmund Freud's Cocaine Years." *New York Times*, July 21, 2011. https://www.nytimes.com/2011/07/24/books/review/an-anatomy-of-addiction-by-howard-markel-book-review.html.

O'Donnell, Mimi, as told to Adam Green. "Mimi O'Donnell Reflects on the Loss of Philip Seymour Hoffman and the Devastation of Addiction." *Vogue*, December 13, 2017. https://www.vogue.com/article/philip-seymour-hoffman-mimi-odonnell-vogue-january-2018-issue.

Oenbrink, Raymond. "What Does Addiction Feel Like? Here's a Clear Picture of What It's Like to Experience Addiction, to Go Through Withdrawal, and to Work Toward Sobriety." Appalachian Wellness, August 10, 2018. https://appwell.net/what-does-addiction-feel-like-heres-a-clear-picture-of-what-its-like-to-experience-addiction-to-go-through-withdrawal-and-to-work-toward-sobriety/

"Opioids and the Brain." PursueCare, April 10, 2019. https://www.pursuecare.com/opioids-and-the-brain/.

Partnership to End Addiction. "First Nationally Accredited Addiction Medicine Residency Programs to Start July." May 2011. https://drugfree.org/drug-and-alcohol-news/first-nationally-accredited-addiction-medicine-residency-programs-to-start-july/.

Pattemore, Chantelle. "How Do Adderall and Meth (Methamphetamine) Differ?" Healthline, January 20, 2023. Medically reviewed by Philip Ngo, PharmD. https://www.healthline.com/health/adhd/how-do-adderall-and-meth-methamphetamine.

Pergolizzi, Joseph, Jo Ann K. LeQuang, and Frank Breve. "The End of the X-Waiver: Not a Moment Too Soon!" *Cureus* 13, no. 5 (May 19, 2021): e15123. doi: 10.7759/cureus.15123. PMID: 34159025; PMCID: PMC8212919. https://pubmed.ncbi.nlm.nih.gov/34159025/.

Bibliography

Physician Specialty Data Report. "ACGME Residents and Fellows with a U.S. Doctor of Medicine (U.S. MD) Degree by Specialty, 2017." Accessed March 24, 2022, https://www.aamc.org/data-reports/workforce/interactive-data/acgme-residents-and-fellows-us-doctor-medicine-us-md-degree-specialty-2017.

Porterfield, Carlie. "These Museums Still Have the Sackler Name Up Despite Opioid Crisis Controversy." *Forbes*, May 29, 2018. https://www.forbes.com/sites/carlieporterfield/2022/02/07/these-museums-still-have-the-sackler-name-up-despite-opioid-crisis-controversy/?sh=405ae6b857d5.

Raman, Ryan. "What Is Kratom Tea, and Is It Safe?" *Healthline Newsletter*, February 27, 2020. Medically reviewed by Jillian Kubala. https://www.healthline.com/nutrition/kratom-tea.

Ranapurwala, Shabbar I., Meghan E. Shanahan, Apostolos A. Alexandridis, Scott K. Proescholdbell, Rebecca B. Naumann, Daniel Edwards, Jr., and Stephen W. Marshall. "Opioid Overdose Mortality Among Former North Carolina Inmates: 2000–2015." *American Journal of Public Health* 108, no. 9 (September 2018): 1207–2213. https://doi.org/10.2105/AJPH.2018.304514.

"Report: Government Not Spending Much on Drug Prevention." CNN, May 28, 2009. https://www.cnn.com/2009/HEALTH/05/28/addiction.costs.

Research Recovery Institute. "How Prevalent Is Recovery from Opioid Use Disorder in the United States, and How Do People Get There?" October 2019. https://www.recoveryanswers.org/research-post/opioid-recovery-prevalence-united-states/.

Rich, Ben A. "Physicians' Legal Duty to Relieve Suffering." *The Western Journal of Medicine* 175, no. 3 (September 2001): 151–152. doi: 10.1136/ewjm.175.3.151. PMID: 11527832; PMCID: PMC1071521.

Richards, Katie. "If Cancer Patients Were Treated Like Addicts: Hard-Hitting PSAs Aim to 'Stop the Shame.'" Adweek.com, March 29, 2017. https://www.adweek.com/brand-marketing/if-cancer-patients-were-treated-like-addicts-hard-hitting-psas-aim-to-stop-the-shame/.

Rose, Emma Jane, Giorgia Picci and Diana H. Fishbien. "Neurocognitive Precursors of Substance Misuse Corresponding to Risk, Resistance, and Resilience Pathways: Implications for Prevention Science." *Frontiers in Society* 10 (June 14, 2019). https://www.frontiersin.org/articles/10.3389/fpsyt.2019.00399/full.

Rosen, Andrew. "Not All Addicts Are Alike." Center for Treatment of Anxiety and Mood Disorders. https://centerforanxietydisorders.com/not-addicts-alike/.

Sadeghi, Parvine, and James P. Zacny, "Anesthesia Is a Risk Factor for Drug and Alcohol Craving and Relapse in Ex-Abusers." *Med Hypotheses* 53, no. 6 (December 1999): 490–96. doi: 10.1054/mehy.1999.0797. PMID: 10687890. https://pubmed.ncbi.nlm.nih.gov/10687890/.

Schwartzapfel, B. "When Going to Jail Means Giving Up the Meds That Saved Your Life." The Marshall Project, January 29, 2019. https://www.themarshallproject.org/2019/01/29/when-going-to-jail-means-giving-up-the-meds-that-saved-your-life.

Shah, Mansi, and Martin R. Huecker. "Opioid Withdrawal." *StatPearls*, January 2023, updated July 21, 2023. https://www.ncbi.nlm.nih.gov/books/NBK526012/.

Shaklee. "The Shaklee Difference—Organic and Beyond." Shaklee.com, January 1, 2023. https://us.shaklee.com/about-us.

Sinha, Rajita. "New Findings on Biological Factors Predicting Addiction Relapse Vulnerability." *Current Psychiatry Reports* 13, no. 5 (October 2011): 398–405. doi: 10.1007/s11920-011-0224-0. PMID: 21792580; PMCID: PMC3674771. https://pubmed.ncbi.nlm.nih.gov/21792580/.

Siu, Eric Y., and Tiffany S. Moon. "Opioid-Free and Opioid-Sparing Anesthesia." *International Anesthesiology Clinics* 58, no. 2 (Spring 2020): 34–41. doi: 10.1097/AIA.0000000000000270. https://pubmed.ncbi.nlm.nih.gov/32004171/.

"6 Benefits of Exercise in Addiction Recovery." Medically reviewed by Nanci Stockwell, LCSW, MBA. The Recovery Village, last updated May 3, 2022.

Smith, D.E. "The Evolution of Addiction Medicine as a Medical Specialty." *AMA Journal of*

Ethics, December 2011, accessed March 13, 2022. https://journalofethics.ama-assn.org/article/evolution-addiction-medicine-medical-specialty/2011-12.

Smith, Mark A., and Wendy J. Lynch. "Exercise as a Potential Treatment for Drug Abuse: Evidence from Preclinical Studies." *Frontiers in Psychiatry* 2 (January 12, 2012): 82. doi: 10.3389/fpsyt.2011.00082. PMID: 22347866; PMCID: PMC3276339.

Splett, Matthew. "Kratom Tea Study Stirs Up New Support for Relieving Opioid Dependence." UF Health, University of Florida Health, October 20, 2020. https://ufhealth.org/news/2020/kratom-tea-study-stirs-new-support-relieving-opioid-dependence.

Stangl, Anne L., Valerie A. Earnshaw, Carmen H. Logie, Wim van Brakel, Leickness C. Simbayi, Iman Barré, and John F. Dovidio. "The Health Stigma and Discrimination Framework: A Global, Crosscutting Framework to Inform Research, Intervention Development, and Policy on Health-Related Stigmas." BMC Medicine, BioMed Central, February 15, 2019. https://bmcmedicine.biomedcentral.com/articles/10.1186/s12916-019-1271-3.

Stewart, Jane. "Review. Psychological and Neural Mechanisms of Relapse." *Philosophical Transactions of the Royal Society of London, Series B, Biological Sciences* 363, no. 1507 (October 12, 2008). https://www.ncbi.nlm.nih.gov/pmc/articles/PMC2607321/.

Stine, Susan M., and T.R. Kosten. "Reduction of Opiate Withdrawal-Like Symptoms by Cocaine Abuse During Methadone and Buprenorphine Maintenance." *American Journal of Drug and Alcohol Abuse* 20, no. 4 (November 1994): 445–58. doi: 10.3109/00952999409109183. PMID: 7832179. https://pubmed.ncbi.nlm.nih.gov/7832179/.

"Suboxone vs. Methadone: How Does Suboxone Compare to Methadone?" American Addiction Centers, January 7, 2022, updated September 15, 2022. https://americanaddictioncenters.org/suboxone/compare.

Substance Abuse and Mental Health Service Administration (SAMHSA). "Buprenorphine." U.S. Department of Health & Human Services, last updated July 18, 2023. https://www.samhsa.gov/medications-substance-use-disorders/medications-counseling-related-conditions/buprenorphine.

Substance Abuse and Mental Health Service Administration (SAMHSA). "Co-Occurring Disorders and Other Health Conditions." U.S. Department of Health & Human Services, January 25, 2023, last updated July 26, 2023. https://www.samhsa.gov/medications-substance-use-disorders/medications-counseling-related-conditions/co-occurring-disorders.

Substance Abuse and Mental Health Service Administration (SAMHSA). "Recovery Housing: Best Practices and Suggested Guidelines." U.S. Department of Health and Human Services. https://www.samhsa.gov/resource/ebp/recovery-housing-best-practices-suggested-guidelines.

Substance Abuse and Mental Health Services Administration (U.S.); Office of the Surgeon General (U.S.). "Chapter 2: The Neurobiology of Substance Use, Misuse, and Addiction." *Facing Addiction in America: The Surgeon General's Report on Alcohol, Drugs, and Health*, November 2016. https://www.ncbi.nlm.nih.gov/books/NBK424849/.

Talchekar, Anjali. "Timeline: A History of Addiction Treatment." Recovery.org, November 29, 2021, updated July 16, 2023. Medically reviewed by Scot Thomas, M.D. https://recovery.org/drug-treatment/history/.

U.S. Department of Health and Human Services. "How Effective Is Drug Addiction Treatment?" National Institutes of Health, June 3, 2020. https://nida.nih.gov/publications/principles-drug-addiction-treatment-research-based-guide-third-edition/frequently-asked-questions/how-effective-drug-addiction-treatment.

U.S. National Library of Medicine. (2021, February 15). "Methadone: MedlinePlus Drug Information." MedlinePlus, last revised May 15, 2023. https://medlineplus.gov/druginfo/meds/a682134.html

Upton, Fred. "Drug Overdose Death Rates. PRESCRIPTION DRUG DIVERSION: COMBATING THE SCOURGE." Subcommittee on Commerce, Manufacturing, and Trade, U.S. House of Representatives, March 1, 2012. energycommerce.house.gov.

Valero, Rose M. "Hearing the Voice of Addiction: A Case Study." Doctoral dissertation, California Institute of Integral Studies, 2021 (Publication No. 28497929). ProQuest, https://www.proquest.com/openview/14fcc88025b72c30823eae8377b1f644/1?pq-origsite=gscholar&cbl=18750&diss=y.

Van Horn, Ngoc L., and Megan Street. "Night Terrors." *StatPearls*, January 2023, last updated May 29, 2023. PMID: 29630274. https://pubmed.ncbi.nlm.nih.gov/29630274/.

Vestal, Christine. "Most Hospital ERs Won't Treat Your Addiction. These Will." The Pew Charitable Trusts, September 21, 2018. https://www.pewtrusts.org/en/research-and-analysis/blogs/stateline/2018/09/21/most-hospital-ers-wont-treat-your-addiction-these-will.

Volkow, Nora. "Making Addiction Treatment More Realistic and Pragmatic: The Perfect Should Not Be the Enemy of the Good." National Institute on Drug Abuse, National Institutes of Health, U.S. Department of Health & Human Services, January 4, 2022. https://nida.nih.gov/about-nida/noras-blog/2022/01/making-addiction-treatment-more-realistic-pragmatic-perfect-should-not-be-enemy-good.

Voss, Janet Piper. "Relapse After Long-Term Sobriety." The Missouri Bar, accessed March 24, 2022. https://mobar.org/site/content/Articles/Addiction/Relapse_After_Long-Term_Sobriety.

Wakeman, Sarah E., Marc R. Larochelle, and Omid Ameli, et al. "Comparative Effectiveness of Different Treatment Pathways for Opioid Use Disorder." *JAMA Network Open* 3, no. 2 (February 5, 2020):e1920622. doi:10.1001/jamanetworkopen.2019.20622.

Walker, Leah. "Opioid Addiction: Why Don't More Rehabs Use Suboxone?" American Addition Centers, updated August 7, 2023. Reviewed by Scot Thomas, M.D. https://rehabs.com/pro-talk/opioid-addiction-treatment-why-dont-more-rehabs-use-suboxone/.

Watson, Stephanie. "Feel-Good Hormones: How They Affect Your Mind, Mood, and Body." Harvard Health, July 20, 2021. https://www.health.harvard.edu/mind-and-mood/feel-good-hormones-how-they-affect-your-mind-mood-and-body.

Wienecke, Elmar, and Claudia Nolden. "Long-Term HRV Analysis Shows Stress Reduction by Magnesium Intake." *MMW Fortschritte der Medizin* 158, Supplement 6 (December 2016). https://pubmed.ncbi.nlm.nih.gov/27933574/.

WVUToday. "WVU Rockefeller Neuroscience Institute First in U.S. to Use Deep Brain Stimulation to Fight Opioid Addiction." November 5, 2019, accessed March 24, 2022. https://wvutoday.wvu.edu/stories/2019/11/05/wvu-rockefeller-neuroscience-institute-first-in-u-s-to-use-deep-brain-stimulation-to-fight-opioid-addiction.

Zuber, Katie, Patricia Stratch, and Elizabeth Pérez-Chiqués. "Five Myths of the Opioid Crisis." Rockefeller Institute of Government, February 7, 2019. https://rockinst.org/blog/five-myths-of-the-opioid-crisis/.

Index

Accreditation Council for Graduate Medical Education (ACGME) 147
ADD 13, 17, 18, 22, 61, 156, 211
Adderall 17, 18, 61
addiction counselor 168
addiction fellowships 44, 133, 247
addictionologist 44, 55, 135, 228, 235, 238
alcoholics 9, 167
Alcoholics Anonymous 166
Allan, Chas 249
Amen, Dr. Daniel 122, 184
American Society of Addiction Medicine (ASAM) 245
anesthesia 44, 115, 128, 129, 133, 136, 142, 177, 197
anesthesiologist 115, 129, 139, 142
Arvidson, Christine 249
Ativan 56
autistic spectrum disorders (ASD) 9

B-complex 17
Barnett, Roger 124, 251
Bartz, Helene 91, 99
benzodiazepines 56, 64
bio-neurological 23, 62, 69, 156, 178, 183, 245
bipolar 22, 23, 107
Bradfield, Jenni 31-34, 90, 93, 96, 100, 216, 239
brain's reward center 17
breakthrough pain 37, 46, 53
Brown, Terry 251
Buchheit, Dr. Thomas 250
buprenorphine 148, 178, 232, 246

Cagel, ZoeAnn 251
Carr, Deryle 131, 151, 251
Cary, Pam 63, 251
CBD oil 209-210, 221
CDC (Centers for Disease Control) 136, 138, 180, 227
Chaney, Dr. Steve 124
childhood schizophrenia 9
chronic disease 4, 68, 166
Clonazepam 63, 221, 227, 230
co-dependency 66

cognitive development 13
controlled substance 43
Controlled Substances Act (CSA) 209
Courney, Yarrow 26, 31-46, 50-54, 72, 120, 175
Crisis Bonding Syndrome 87

Daggy, Dr. Bruce 251
DEA 3, 5, 47, 51
denial 5, 9, 19, 23, 70, 75, 78, 86, 150, 156
Depakote 22
detox 15, 22, 24, 40, 44, 59-62, 82-84, 88, 106, 138, 151, 164, 179, 228
Diagnostic and Statistical Manual of Mental Disorders (DSM) 8-9
doctor shopping 62
dopamine 18, 22, 80, 92, 187, 219, 232
drug dependency 3, 22-23, 42, 55, 67-69, 92, 106, 146, 194, 200
dual diagnosis 60, 108, 148, 166-168, 243, 246
Duke 127, 169, 150

emotional trauma 9, 53
endorphins 110, 116, 187, 217, 221
Estes, Dr. Rebecca 42-57, 115, 132-135, 222, 249
Ewing, Katherine 251

FDA 21, 47, 126
fentanyl 32, 139, 240-247
fifth vital sign 37
Fine, Marjorie 251
Foran, Tom 249
functional alcoholic 9, 93

GAD (general anxiety disorder) 22
Gant, Dr. Charles 121
Glacken, Jennifer 251
Gorski, Moyra 163, 251
Gould, Janie 251
Gupta, Dr. Arun 121, 245-248, 250

Hage, John 251
Haloperidol 17

Index

Hart, Wanda 156, 251
heroin 47, 138, 178, 181, 235
Herrick, James 250
high tolerance 4, 9, 43, 92–93, 128–129, 136, 142, 148, 182, 238
HIPPA 49, 57, 177
Hippocratic Oath 46, 159
hitting bottom 107, 214

intestinal blockage 157–158

Johnson, Marcia Shephard 251

Kennecke, Angela 1–2, 251
Ketamine 34, 140, 142
Kilby, Susan 249
kratom tea 158–159, 161, 180, 235

lithium 23

magnesium 17
Marsh, Katherine 251
MAT (medicine assisted therapy) 167, 251
McManus, Dr. Jamie 251
MDMA (methylenedioxymethamphetamine) 230
mental health disorders 7–8, 135, 148, 226, 251
methadone 75–76, 136–138, 144–148, 158–162, 177–179, 232, 447
methamphetamine 18
moral defect 169
morphine 34, 36, 51, 102, 140–142, 158–160, 177–178, 180, 231
motor tics 17
MOUD (medications for opioid use disorder) 68, 148, 155, 179, 243, 246, 248
Moules, Pam Sugarman 251

Naloxone 138, 246
Naltrexone 148
Narcan 138–139, 246, 248
Narcotics Anonymous 60, 68, 79, 91, 122, 154–155, 166, 179, 188, 229, 243
NASM (National Academy of Sports Medicine) 167
NDE (near death experience) 114, 240
neurological disorders 13, 17, 22–23, 30, 62, 69, 149, 178–179, 185, 245
neurologist 53, 174
neuropathways 16
neurotransmitters 17, 187
NGE-tube nasogastric tube 158–160, 177
night terrors 12–13, 225, 235
nutritional support 121, 149, 185

OCD 13, 22
Omegas 49
opioid antagonist 24
out of network 45, 80

oxytocin 187
Oxycontin 1, 19, 21, 36–37, 41, 47, 53, 55, 74, 156
Oxycontin Express 58

pain management 37, 41, 46, 48, 57–59, 115, 132, 135, 144, 147, 250
Paschal, Worth 10, 25, 98, 113, 119, 151, 205, 233, 250
Percocet 21–22, 42, 312–135
personal boundaries 66
Peterson, Caryl 95, 107, 131, 251
Phenobarbital 164
Pill Mills 47, 57, 247
Portenoy, Dr. Russell K. 47
precursors of addiction 3, 8, 30, 243
"Prescription Drug Diversion: Combatting the Scourge" 58
Propofol 31
psychiatric hospital 6–9, 17, 44, 167, 180–181, 187
psychiatrist 8, 22–23, 44, 135, 227, 229, 231
psychoactive drug 8
psychologist 23, 28, 53
PTSD (Post Traumatic Syndrome Disorder) 39, 53–56, 63, 92, 115, 133, 142, 148, 168, 174, 182, 194, 197, 229
puberty 13, 20
public policy 8, 24, 173, 179, 211, 215, 242–243
Purdue Pharma 3, 19, 21, 37, 46

rehab 39, 44, 56, 59, 64, 84, 96, 150–151, 184
residential program 67
respiratory depression 56
Ross, Justin 249

Sackler family 19, 46
Scheider, Daniel 251
Schivito, Brenda Richards 251
self-medicating 9, 120, 194, 203
Serenity Prayer 74, 98
Seroquel 23, 164
Serotonin 22, 196
Shaklee 16, 49, 58, 60, 89, 101, 120, 124, 209
Sims, Lu 251
Sobriety House 77, 90–94, 107, 109–110, 153–154, 159, 164–166
sociopathic personality disorder 9
SPECT (single photon emission computed tomography) 122
Strickland, Cynthia 251
suboxone 3, 24–25, 41, 43, 55–57, 59, 81, 84–87, 122, 131, 138, 148, 158–159, 162, 177–179, 228–230, 235, 242–248
substance abuse counselor 19, 150, 155, 168
SUD (substance use disorder) 3, 61–63, 69, 159, 167–168, 179, 242, 244–245, 250

Taylor, Jacob 112, 120, 122–124, 157, 189, 193–194, 205–206, 249

Index

THC 209–210
Thompson, Tom 174, 249
Tourette's Syndrome 17, 48, 61
Twelve Steps 90, 92, 107, 150, 155, 168, 198

Valium 56, 312
vocal tics 17

Wright, Torin 251

X-waiver 3, 24, 81, 84, 159
Xanax 48, 55, 56, 61, 163